Lower Urinary Tract Obstruction in Childhood

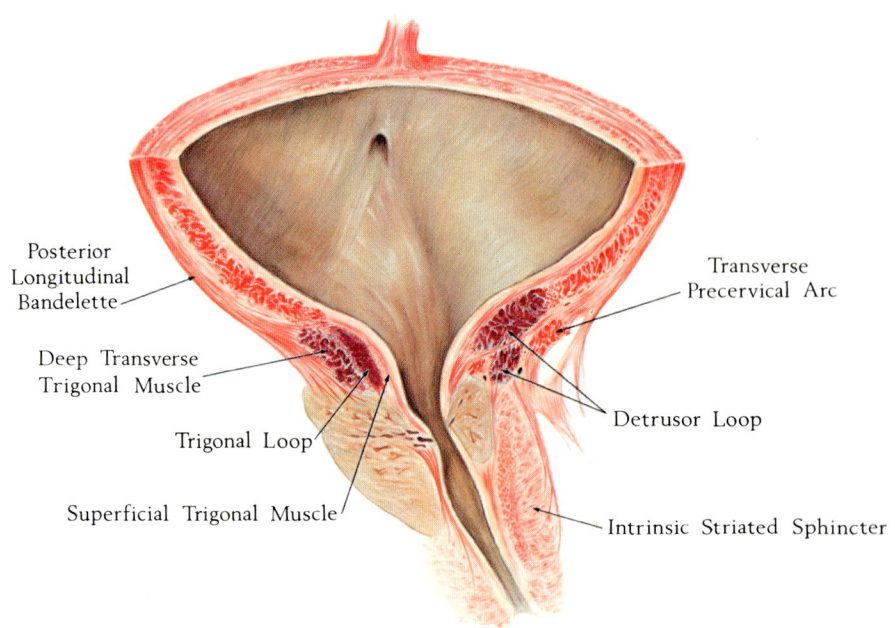

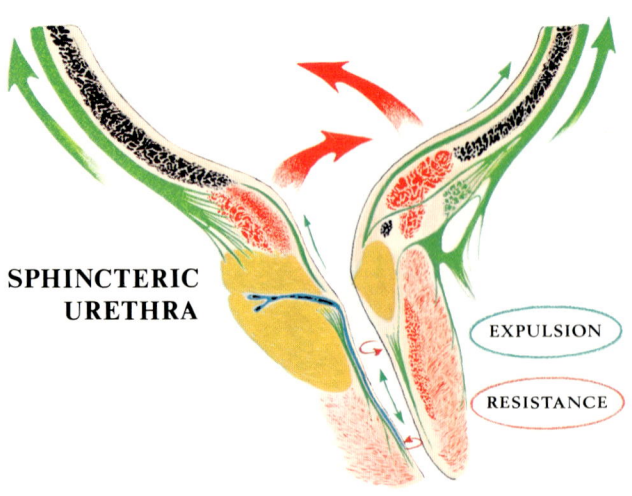

Principal histotopographic musculature of the male sphincteric urethra and its implied function.

BRADFORD WOODBRIDGE YOUNG, M.D.
*Attending Urologist, Children's Hospital of San Francisco
Senior Research Member
Institute of Medical Sciences
Pacific Medical Center, San Francisco*

Lower Urinary Tract Obstruction in Childhood

With Illustrations by
JAMES W. BRODALE

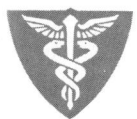

LEA & FEBIGER · 1972 · PHILADELPHIA

ISBN 0-8121-0381-5

Copyright © 1972 by Lea & Febiger. Copyright under the International Copyright Union. All Rights Reserved. This book is protected by copyright. No part of it may be reproduced in any manner or by any means without written permission from the publisher.

Published in Great Britain by Henry Kimpton Publishers, London

Library of Congress Catalog Card Number: 72-175467

Printed in the United States of America

*This book is dedicated
to*
Professor Salvador Gil Vernet
*Anatomist, Urologist, Philosopher
"Le Maître"*

Preface

The subject to be investigated is that of the child with difficult urination who, upon examination, shows signs of obstruction to the outflow of urine from the bladder.

There is reason to believe that this is a specific problem unrelated to urinary obstruction in the adult. It has embryological implications, as well as anatomical ones. It carries a much graver import of severe renal damage, and is considerably more difficult to correct than acquired urinary tract obstruction in the adult.

Many of the difficulties surrounding the problem of outflow obstruction to the lower urinary tract in children have arisen from the lack of a clear definition of the nature of the obstruction and from confusion about the normal anatomy and function of the sphincteric urethra.

The undertaking of this critical review of infravesical obstruction in childhood has entailed the sorting out of observations, conclusions, attitudes and myths. Rather than finding that all congenital lower urinary tract obstructive disease has a common cause, it is evident that at least twelve distinct entities, often in combination, present the clinical appearance of "vesical neck obstruction." To arrive at this conclusion, it has been necessary to restudy carefully the current concepts of the embryology, anatomy and physiology of the urinary bladder, and to incorporate into a coherent pattern the recent advances in the hydrodynamics of urinary flow, cineradiography and smooth-muscle function.

The chief value of this study, from the clinical standpoint, is to provide a more accurate criterion for the selection of children who will benefit from surgical intervention, while more securely identifying those in whom expectant management and maturation can be anticipated to balance the sphincteric functions of the lower urinary tract.

The principles which are described suggest a host of possibilities for the imaginative development of further surgical and medical procedures, for which there is an urgent need. Some of these are immediately evident and could be easily adopted; others, more subtle, may require years of technical refinement at ultrastructural, genetic and molecular levels before they can be applied clinically.

As this study unfolded, it was interesting to discover that some of the ancient myths were true, some of the conclusions erroneous, some of the attitudes derivative and expedient, but that the clinical and pathological observations, for the most part, were all extraordinarily accurate.

To Dr. Wyland H. Leadbetter, who first set me this Jason's fleece to pursue, I should like to express my most profound gratitude.

BRADFORD WOODBRIDGE YOUNG, M.D.

San Francisco, California

Acknowledgments

I would like to express my deep appreciation to those who have helped me in the preparation of this monograph.

The hospitality and generous access to the libraries, laboratories and hospitals afforded me by my British and European colleagues during my Reisejahr in 1965 account for much of the broadened point of view of this study. I hope that my response to this stimulation and interest will be evident in this book.

All of the serially sectioned embryological specimens were prepared by Mrs. Loretta Blake, who established and managed the histological laboratory. Mr. Kenneth Benjamin was of great assistance in preparing the celloidin sections. Photographic reproductions of the original photomicrographs and of Mr. James Brodale's drawings were expertly made by Mr. Sam Ehrlich, Mr. Proctor Jones and Mr. Thomas Moulin. Mrs. Norma Bevans managed the many details of the laboratory research program, collected and recorded the data, and patiently prepared the finished manuscript.

Dr. Harold K. Faber, Emeritus Professor of Pediatrics at the Stanford University School of Medicine, has not only taught, encouraged and wisely counseled me for many years but, in addition, kindly allowed me the use of his compendious personal file of the pediatric literature.

My wife, from the inception of this study, has enthusiastically encouraged, questioned, rephrased, retyped—and renewed the author.

I would particularly like to thank Mrs. Katherine Wigmore Eyre for making possible the preparation of additional anatomical drawings, which add much clarity to these difficult concepts.

This study was supported in part by Grants 1 R01 HD02041 and HD04117 from the National Institute of Child Health and Human Development, United States Public Health Service.

B. W. Y.

Contents

I. Introduction	1
II. Anatomy of the Bladder and Sphincteric Urethra	11
Development (Embryology)	11
Anatomical Relations	19
Musculature of the Bladder and Sphincteric Urethra	23
Gross Anatomy	23
Histotopographic Anatomy	30
Microscopic Anatomy	55
III. Physiology of Micturition	64
Muscular Mechanisms of Urination	64
Neuromuscular Mechanisms	73
Cellular Morphology of Smooth Muscle	76
Hydrodynamics	85
IV. Pathology of Congenital Obstructive Lesions	93
Urethral Valves	97
Fibroelastosis	116
Vesical-Neck Hypertrophy	120
Urethral Polyps	122
Urethral Diverticulum	125
Cysts	126
Cowper's-duct Cysts	126

Müllerian-duct Cysts	128
Megacystis	130
Vesical Dysplasia	141
The Triad ("Prune Belly") Syndrome	141
Sphincteric Hypotonia	143
Neurogenic Bladder	146
Inflammatory Obstruction	149
Urethral Meatal Stenosis	149
Tumor	150
V. Management	**152**
Diagnosis	152
Diagnostic Investigation	155
Treatment	159
Further Considerations	161
VI. Bibliography	**168**
Index	191

I
Introduction

The purposes of this clinicopathological study are to identify the various types of congenital urethral obstruction in the human on an anatomical or embryological basis and to compare these findings with the normal histotopography of the infant urethra.

The material upon which these findings and hypotheses are based includes 3,469 significant serial sections from 26 normal embryos, fetuses, newborns and one 5-year-old child (Table 1). There were four necropsy specimens with obstructive lesions from which 1,187 significant serial sections were obtained and 60 biopsies from 33 surgical cases in children with various congenital obstructive lesions.

Light microscopy study of the specimens was carried out to trace the development of the smooth muscle-bundle structure, collagen, elastic tissue, nerve and ganglion cell distribution in the human urinary bladder and sphincteric urethra. The sections were examined at magnifications of 10 to 1,000 diameters. The distribution and orientation of the sections are shown in Figure 1. Sections made at 6, 8 and 10 to 15 micra (μ) were embedded in either paraffin, rubber-wax or celloidin and stained with Heidenhain-Mallory azan-orange G, Verhoeff-van Gieson, hematoxylin and eosin, Luxol fast-blue-PAS,

TABLE 1. *Development of the Human Sphincteric Urethra Distribution of 3,469 Serial Sections*

No.	Lab Spec. No.	C.R. Length mm	Age	Sex	No. of Sections	Plane
1	Y-2-66	4 mm	(4 weeks)	—	99	Sagittal
2	Y-90-69	9 mm	↑	—	198	Sagittal
3	Y-41-67	11 mm	↓	—	87	Sagittal
4	Y-53-67	20 mm	(8 weeks)	—	172	Sagittal
5	Y-3-66	22 mm	↑	—	200	Horizontal
6	Y-1-66	23 mm		—	93	Sagittal
7	Y-29-67	26 mm		M	282	Sagittal
8	Y-51-67	45 mm		M	183	Frontal
9	Y-4-66	50 mm		M	126	Horizontal
10	Y-12-66	50 mm	↓	M	54	Sagittal
11	Y-5-66	55 mm	(12 weeks)	M	114	Sagittal
12	Y-73-68	60 mm	↑	M	180	Frontal
13	Y-35-67	90 mm		F	107	Sagittal
14	Y-7B-66	110 mm		F	282	Horizontal
15	Y-48-67	117 mm	↓	F	120	Sagittal
16	Y-9-66	118 mm	(16 weeks)	M	19	Sagittal
17	Y-49-67	130 mm	↑	M	79	Sagittal
18	Y-61-68	150 mm		M	206	Oblique Frontal
19	Y-55-68	165 mm	↓	M	300	Sagittal
20	Y-8A-66	170 mm	5 months	M	50	Sagittal
		Weight				
21	Y-33-67	1300 gm	5 months	M	230	Horizontal
22	Y-30-67	1300 gm	6 months	F	19	Horizontal
23	Y-15-66	—	8 months	F	20	Sagittal
24	Y-32-67	1690 gm	9 months	M	16	Frontal
25	Y-62-68	Neonate	6 days	M	75	Sagittal
26	Y-BH-66	Child	5 years	M	158	Horizontal
Total Sections					3,469	

Luxol fast-blue-Holmes' silver, PTAH and methyl blue-acid fuchsin (G. Herovici).

The smallest embryo in this series was 4 mm crown-rump (C.R.) length; the series includes one 6-day-old male neonate and one 5-year-old male. There were 15 male specimens and 5 female specimens. There were 6 embryos smaller than 23 mm of indeterminate gonadal sex. Twenty specimens were under 170 mm C.R. length (i.e., 5 months) and 4 fetuses were 5, 6, 8 and 9 months respectively.

Whole mount sections of the bladder, rectum, sphincteric urethra and perineum were made in sagittal, coronal, horizontal (transverse) and oblique frontal planes to demonstrate specific features of muscle-

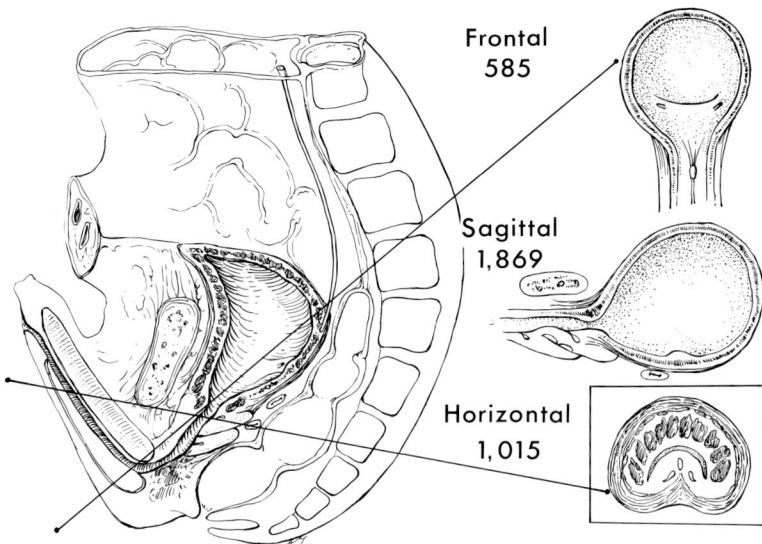

FIG. 1. Planes of 3,469 microscopic sections (6-10 μ) in the human embryo and fetus.

bundle structure, collagen and elastic elements, ganglia, nerve and duct system distribution.[507,25,147,510]

Muscle-bundle groupings, distribution and relations in the developing embryo and fetus were described in detail and were then mapped by individual drawings from the microscopic sections. In addition, Ektachrome transparencies were made of significant serial groupings and redisplayed by rapid automatic projection to trace the course of the muscle bundles, nerves and pertinent ducts. The developing duct systems traced included müllerian, mesonephric, ureter, vas deferens and Cowper's (Bartholin's). Differences in the maturation of the pelvic urogenital sinus were traced in a similar manner with particular attention to the urethrovaginal folds. A readily reproducible muscle-bundle, collagen and elastic pattern was established in this material.

Four children with lower urinary tract obstructive disease coming to autopsy were investigated by the same methods as the normal controls. There were 4 males, 2 of whom were stillborn, one 3 years old and one 9 years old (Table 2). In the case of the 3-year-old male with congenital bulbomembranous urethral obstruction, 527 transverse serial sections were made from the sphincteric urethra and bladder

TABLE 2. *Obstruction of Sphincteric Urethra Distribution of 1157 Serial Sections*

	Patient	Source	Age	Sex	No. of Sections	Plane	Pathological Diagnosis
1	U.A.	Stillborn	0 yrs	M	420	Horizontal	Valves + cloacal membrane dysplasia
2	B.H.	Stillborn	0 yrs	M	200	Horizontal	Bulbomembranous stenosis
3	M.C.	Autopsy	3 yrs	M	527	Horizontal	Bulbomembranous stenosis + vesical neck
4	G.V.	Autopsy	9 yrs	M	10	Horizontal	Cowper's duct cysts

neck, extending from the bulbomembranous junction through the midportion of the trigone.

In a stillborn with aplasia of the penis, cloacal membrane failure and atresia of the urethra with associated urethral valves, 420 sections were obtained of the entire bladder from the area of urethral atresia to the deformed urachal remnant. In a 9-year-old with congenital obstruction of the urethra due to Cowper's duct cysts, 10 whole-mount celloidin step sections were obtained,* and in another stillborn with bulbomembranous urethral obstruction 200 sections were obtained.

Biopsy material was obtained from 33 patients, ranging in age from 6 days to 67 years (Table 3). Specimens were obtained from

*Patient of S. Gil Vernet.

TABLE 3. *Obstruction of Sphincteric Urethra Clinicopathological Diagnoses (Biopsies)*

Diagnosis	No.
Vesical Neck Obstruction	8
Megacystis	5
Urethral Stenosis	3
Exstrophy	1
Triad Syndrome	1
Valves	3
Hypertrophy (?)	6
Neurogenic	4
Interstitial Cystitis	2

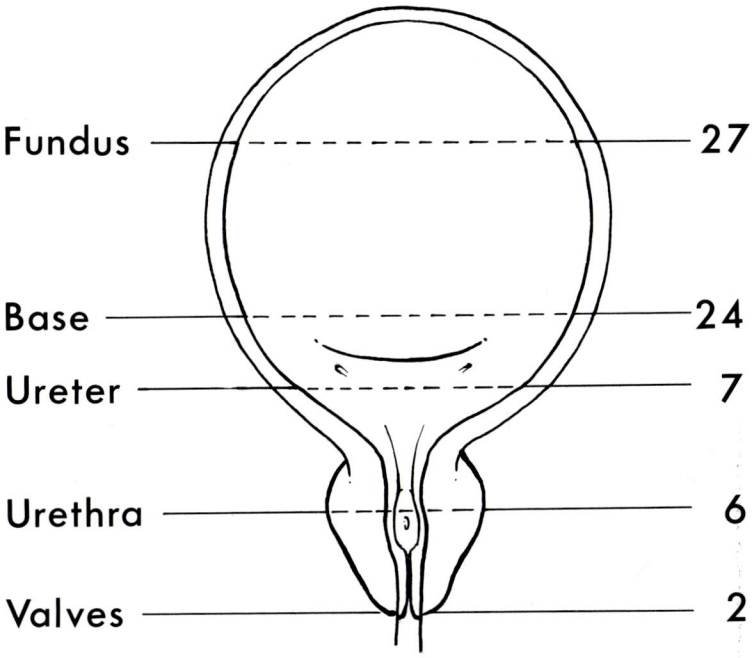

FIG. 2. Distribution of 60 biopsy sites (33 patients).

the bladder, vesical neck and proximal urethra, as well as the inframontane urethra, and included portions of valves removed at surgery in two cases (Fig. 2). This portion of the study was initiated to confirm some of the pathological changes in smooth muscle, connective tissue and elastic layers of the bladder neck and urethra, and also to serve as an indicator of age-specific variations in the microscopic structure of the detrusor muscle and vesical neck. Step sections of the entire adult female urethra were obtained from autopsy material in two cases.

The history of vesical neck obstruction has been intimately related to the description of the musculature of the vesical neck and sphincteric urethra.[535,520,329,312,218,133,91] It has also been widely discussed in relation to chronic inflammatory processes of the cranial prostate. In the older literature little differentiation was made between vesical neck obstruction in adults and in children. That there might be several different types with different etiologies was largely discounted in the search for a common etiology. All that "idiopathic vesical neck obstruction" signified in the different age groups was the absence of any obviously obstructing prostatic adenoma. Borm and Clausen,[32] in an exceedingly thorough review of the world literature, credit Fuller in 1897[164] with the first description of sclerotic vesical neck obstruction in adults, though the French urologists were searching for some cause of this apparent obstruction as early as 1850 (Civale). Guthrie in 1834[197] described the condition in an article entitled "On the bar at the neck of the bladder." Marion in 1933[338] was the first to make an attempt to separate the several clinically evident types. Marion also struggled with the concept of urethral valves, detrusor atony and megacystis, as noted in the preamble to his description:

> "Il y a longtemps que les urologists ont eu l'attention attirée par des retentions d'urine plus ou moins complètes d'une origine très difficile a dèmonstrer. La lésion provocatrice n'apparaisant nettement ni du côté de l'urétere ni du côté de la véssie. Mércier en 1884 incriminait des valvules situées au niveau du col. Civale, en 1850, pensait qu'il s'agissait d'une atonie de la véssie. Cette théorie de l'atonie vesicale fût soutenue et vulgarisée en 1889 par Guyon qui a créc le nom "Prostatisme sans prostate" et cette théorie fût admise pendant de nombreuses années. En 1922 je mettais en doute l'éxistence de ces soi-disant 'prostatiques'."[339]

His classification of the "Maladie du Col Vesical" was as follows:

1. Hypertonicity of the internal sphincter (absence of histological lesions—normal muscular fibers).
2. Hypertrophied muscle fibers with no other associated pathological lesion involved.
3. Inflammatory infiltration and sclerosis of muscle and the mucosa.
4. Inflammatory infiltration and fibrosis associated with a glandular proliferation.

Obstruction to the outflow of urine at the bladder neck without apparent cause has been described under many names: Prostatisme sans prostate (Guyon[198]), dysectasié du col vesical (Legueu et Dossot[313]), maladie du col vesicale (Marion[338]), Marion's disease (Nanson,[370] Bodian[27]), cervicite cronica plastica sclerotica (Lasio), median bar (Randell,[424] H. H. Young[562]), contracture of the vesical neck (Chetwood,[87] Caulk,[80] Nesbit and Crenshaw[377]), annulussklerose (Praetorius[413]), idiopathisch sphinkterhypertonie (Rubritius[445]), contracture of the bladder neck (Beer[17]), vesical neck obstruction, Caulk's disease (Trabucco, et al.[502]), dysfunction of the bladder neck (Thompson, G. J.[497]).

These concepts have all been applied to lower urinary tract obstruction in infants and children, despite the fact that the etiological and anatomical terms are frequently misleading.

Campbell[74] demonstrated submucous fibrosis in specimens removed from the vesical neck in children. Gross, Randolph and Wise[194] were unable to demonstrate any predictable pathology in their series of cases. Some specimens showed inflammatory changes, some fibrosis, and others revealed no specific pathology. Bodian[27] presented an attractive theory of "fibroelastosis" based upon his findings of an increased amount of elastic tissue in the sphincteric urethra. He proposed this possibly congenital abnormality as the underlying cause of the obstruction.

Legueu[313] thought that contracture of the vesical neck in adults was a generalized hypertrophy of all tissue elements and could exist without inflammatory changes or new gland formation. This hypothesis would correspond to that of Marion's first two groups.

Rubritius and Schwartz[444] recognized a sclerosis of the muscular internal sphincter and attributed the obstruction to this. Von Lichtenberg[517] admitted the sclerosis but attributed it to an underlying prostatitis which had secondarily invaded the sphincter. This corresponds to Marion's second and third groups, although Marion felt that the sclerosis was secondary to urethral infection rather than prostatic in origin.

Pisani[403] considered that sclerosis of the vesical neck was secondary to infection but went further in proposing a hereditary predisposition to the sclerosis as a local or systemic response to infection, particularly neisserian infection. He based this on the clinical observation that contracture was often seen in the antecedents of the patient. This was perhaps a more sociological than anatomical observation but not without merit, inasmuch as a certain type of "fibroelastosis" of the bladder neck appears now to be congenital and familial.

Chwalla,[90] in examining biopsies of the vesical neck, encountered edema of the mucosa and chronic inflammatory infiltration, but did not observe hypertrophy of the vesical neck musculature, or fibrosis, and deduced that the cause of the rigidity was obscure.

Alken[3] has considered a constitutional degeneration of connective tissue as a cause, and H. H. Young, Frontz and Baldwin[563] proposed the concept of congenital urethral valves.

Glingar[188] spoke of the presence of "semi-valvules" with their concavities directed against the urinary stream to account for the apparent obstruction. He could not demonstrate this cystoscopically and Marion[337] claimed that there was no anatomical basis for this finding.

S. Gil Vernet[175] has not encountered valvular structures either in patients or at autopsy. He does not deny the possibility that they exist, but has stated that they must be rare. Gil Vernet found no cases of hypertrophy of the musculature of the vesical neck, though he found fibrosclerosis of the muscle fibers of the internal sphincter in adults and felt that this was secondary to an inflammatory process which was primary in the submucosal glands of the vesical neck or arose from the cranial prostate.

The possibility has been suggested (Dossot and Fey) that the vesical neck syndrome was a functional one and did not have an anatomical basis.

Marion[337,338] compared *congenital* hypertrophy of the vesical neck to congenital pyloric stenosis and flatly stated that it was smooth-muscle hypertrophy of the vesical neck. He also postulated the congenital absence of smooth-muscle fibers at the vesical neck, which he described as the "dilatory" ones. These he described as probably the vesicocervical fibers of Versari. Gil Vernet was unable to confirm the absence of these fibers in any of his studies.

Throughout this controversy runs the disquieting thread of posterior urethral valves in the male, described by Morgagni as early as 1751.[356] Langenbeck in 1802[291] described urethral valves in his treatise on lithotomy. Velpeau in 1832,[508] in the course of urethral dissection, also reported the presence of these mucosal folds. L'Egenbrodt in 1891 observed posterior urethral "folds" in the course of a cystotomy, and postulated an obstructive role for them. The obstructing posterior urethral valve then entered a stormy political life, proposed alternatively as the only obstructive lesion or as nonexistent, by numerous European urologists.

H. H. Young, Frontz and Baldwin[563] and H. H. Young and McKay[566] established a stylized set of valves in the United States in 1919, and the great valve controversy continued unabated. The difficulty with this diagnosis was that valves were exceedingly difficult to identify clinically, radiographically, and even at autopsy. Their identification has therefore always been, clinically, somewhat suspect. Some descriptions are of large "sails," "demi-valvules" or ridges both superior and inferior to the verumontanum and strictures or diaphragms located anywhere from the bulbous urethra to the vesical neck. In some cases of evident obstruction there was nothing to be identified at all. Significantly, however, the transurethral endoscopic approach for removal of these poorly defined structures with small resectoscopes has brought about clinical cures and the restoration of a normal appearance to voiding cinecystourethrograms in numerous cases.[425,467,256,75]

Pagano[388] credits Tolmaltschew in 1870[500] with the first rational hypothesis for valvular obstruction. In this hypothesis the normal inframontane mucosal plicae, if they were somewhat larger than normal, were thought to trap urine behind them during urination. The intra-urethral pressure behind this riffle was thought capable of producing progressive distention of the fold to produce a valve. Bonnet[28] complained that this explanation did not account for the presence of muscular tissue within the valve. Bazy in 1903[15] felt that valves represented residual folds of the urogenital (cloacal) membrane. The main support for this theory came from the observation that the main site of valve formation was *close* to the junction of the anterior and posterior urethras. The presence of muscle tissue within the valve was accounted for by the development of mesenchymal elements from the urogenital diaphragm. Länger,[289] in 1910, felt that the plicae colliculi represented embryological rests of the müllerian duct. Lowsley[322] agreed that a disturbance of the wolffian or müllerian systems might account for this appearance. Bracci[44] in 1938, Dell'Adami[110] and Pagano[388] are in accord with Tolmaltschew, although Pagano does not discount the theories of Bonnet and Bazy.

The muscular anatomy of the bladder and sphincteric urethra has suffered as much confusion as have its pathological changes. Kohlrausch[280] in 1854, in studying the urinary sphincter, described the *ventral striated musculature* of the sphincteric urethra and also made note of an *external coat of longitudinal (smooth muscle) fibers* which he felt opened the bladder neck. It was Henle, in 1866,[221] who first applied the term "sphincter vesicae internus" to the bladder neck. Waldeyer later concurred in this "lissosphincter,"[519,520] and Heiss, in 1915,[220] laid the anatomical foundation of the concept of the internal sphincter as an *anteriorly placed loop of vesical musculature partially surrounding the vesical neck*. Disse,[117] Peterfi[398] and von Ludinghausen[518] visualized the sphincter internus as being composed of the intersection of two loops of the detrusor musculature. One of these loops was the *sphincter trigonalis* of Versari[509] (1897), Kalischer[259] (1900) and S. Gil Vernet,[171] and the opposing one the *lissosphincter* of Heiss. Hennig[223] pointed out that these two loops were continuations of the detrusor muscle. Rubritius,[445] Hennig[223] and Länger-Toldt,[290] separately, measured the muscle "sphincter internus" (Heiss) as being 1 cm high and 0.5 cm thick. Hennig and Kraft affirmed that the "sphincter internus" alone was responsible for resting continence within the bladder. Kalischer demonstrated that the anterior semilunar fiber bundle drew the bladder neck downward and backward against the vesical neck, a view supported by Zangmeister.[568]

It is not surprising that this ventral arc should have attracted so much attention. It is easily demonstrable upon gross dissection. This is the same arc described by Henle[221] (1866), McCrea,[365] Barkow[12] (1858), von Lüdinghausen,[518] Martius,[343] H. H. Young and Wesson,[565] Eberth[124] Pettigrew[401] and Gomez-Oliveros.[189] H. H. Young and Wesson called it the "external arcuate muscle" and McCrea labeled it the "external vesical sphincter." Uhlenhuth[506] called it quite directly the "ventral loop of the detrusor longitudinal muscle." S. Gil Vernet, in his *Biologia y Patologia de la Prostata*[170,171,172] and in the recently published "Morphology and Function of Vesico-Prostato-Urethral Musculature,"[176] describes in full detail the histotopographic anatomy of the muscle-bundle structure of the sphincteric urethra and has provided a definitive correlation of the literature with his own monumental investigations.

II
Anatomy of the Bladder and Sphincteric Urethra

In this description, an attempt will be made to focus sharply upon established events and principles of the embryology and morphology of the bladder and proximal urethra. The anatomy requires recapitulation and clarification to serve as basis for a clear understanding of the normal mechanism of urination.

Development (Embryology)

The cloaca, that part of the hind gut lying caudal to the allantoic stalk, is divided into an anterior portion, the *primitive urogenital sinus*, and a posterior portion, the *rectum*. The septum dividing the two chambers is the *urorectal septum*. This is formed by a fold of the wall of the entodermal cloaca which grows caudally to fuse with the primitive cloacal membrane in the 8-mm fetus. The posterior portion of the cloacal membrane becomes the *anal membrane*, and the ventral or anterior portion the *urogenital membrane*. The urogenital membrane perforates before the anal membrane (13-mm to 16-mm embryo). The primitive urogenital sinus forms the bladder, primary urethra, and urogenital sinus proper[405,206] (Fig. 3).

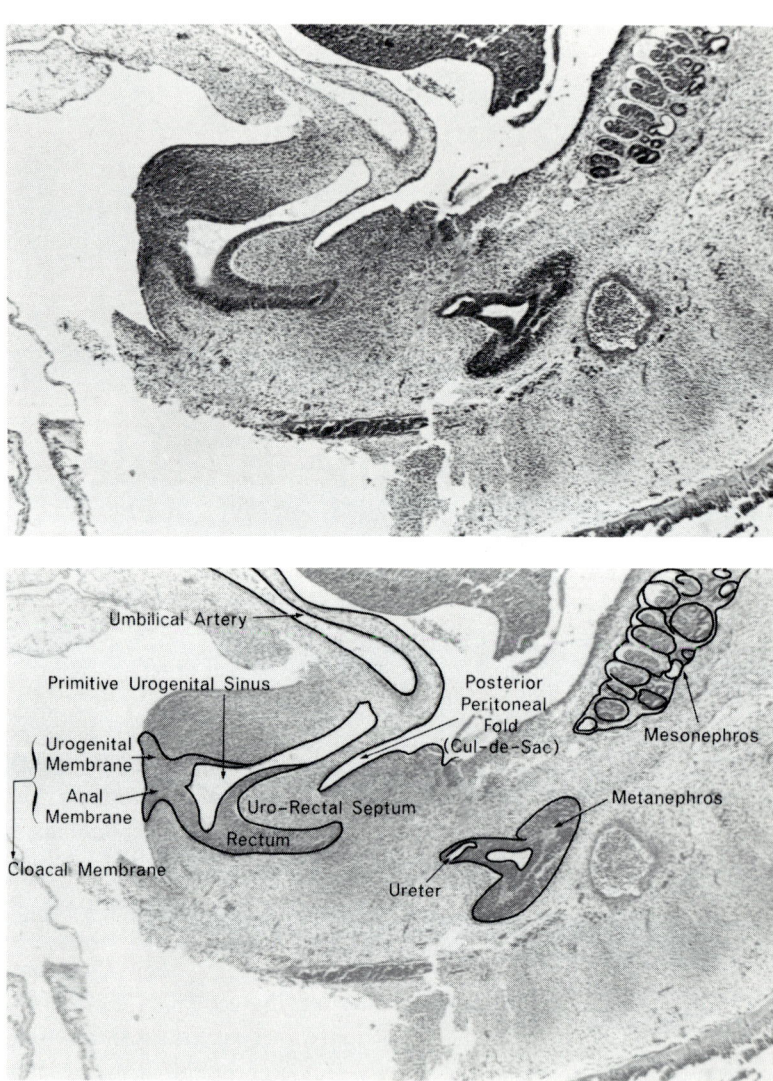

FIG. 3. 8-mm human embryo to show relations of urorectal septum to primitive urogenital sinus and the cloacal membrane. Sagittal section. Note the extent of the cloacal epithelium along the dorsal wall of the primitive urogenital sinus. Original magnification X40.

The mesonephric (wolffian) ducts which originally open into the undivided primitive cloaca at the 4.2-mm stage become incorporated into the posterior wall of the urorectal septum (Fig. 4).

In the 5- to 6-mm embryo, the ureteral buds from the mesonephric

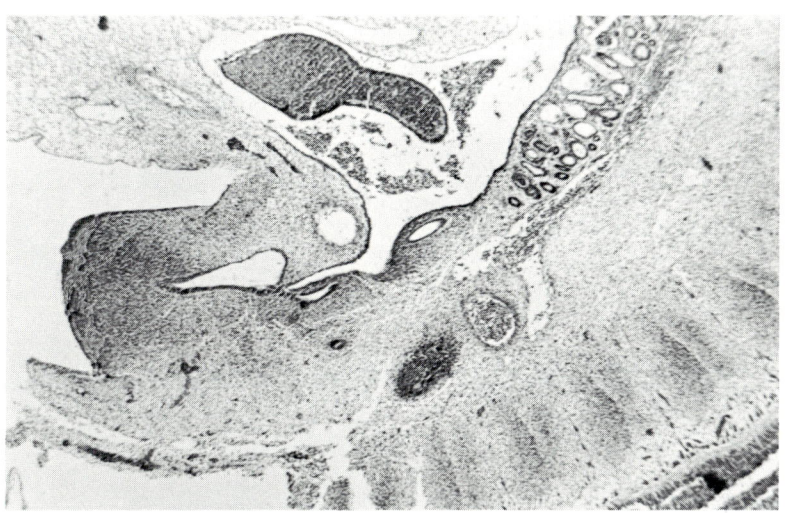

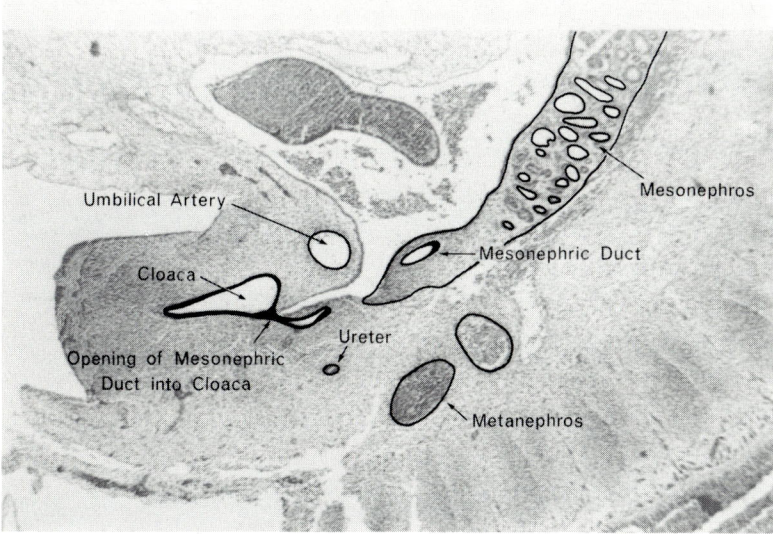

FIG. 4. 8-mm human embryo to show relations of mesonephric duct to cloaca, ureter and metanephros at this stage. Parasagittal section. Original magnification X40.

duct appear and, as their terminal ends migrate cephalad to definitive sites on the posterior wall of the urogenital sinus, the progressive widening of the terminal segment of the conjoined mesonephric duct is presumed to be incorporated into the posterior wall of the urogenital

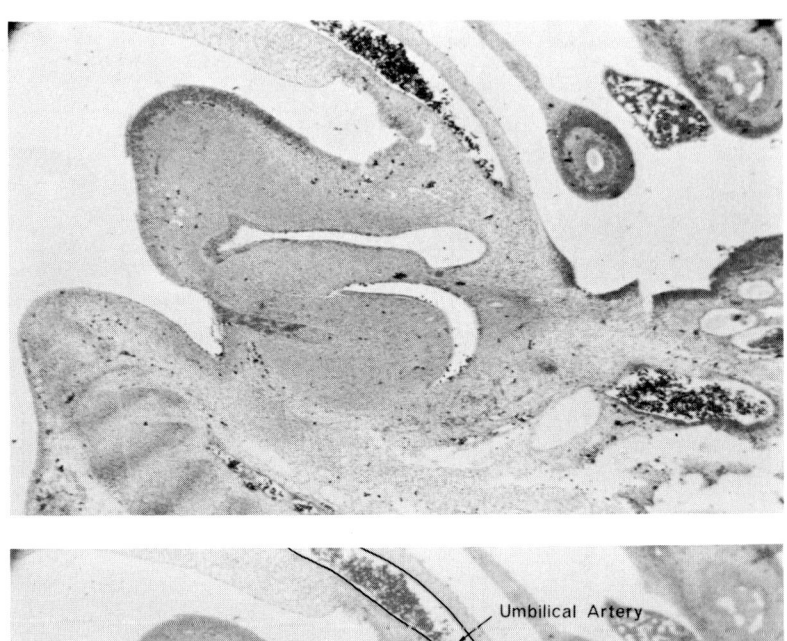

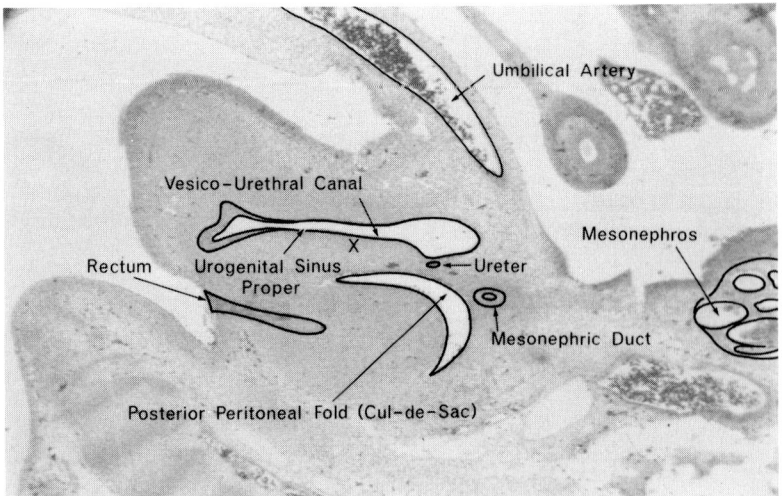

FIG. 5. 20-mm embryo. Parasagittal section to show vesicourethral canal, constriction marking future vesical neck, and *urogenital sinus proper*. The opening of the mesonephric duct into the urogenital sinus (not in this plane of section) is indicated by the sign X. Original magnification X40.

sinus as the *trigone*. Since the mesonephric ducts are of mesodermal origin, this portion of the bladder is usually considered to be mesodermal.[531, 8, 394, 25]

Gruenwald[195] has pointed out the interdependence of the müllerian and wolffian duct systems in their development, in which the wolffian duct plays the leading role. The separation of the ureter from the wolffian duct is the subject of some speculation. Gyllensten (1949),[199] Williams (1951)[536] and Frazer[159] postulate an incorporation into the posterior wall of the urogenital sinus of the intervening portion of the common duct with subsequent desquamation of a portion of its wall to bring about its obliteration. Bengmark (1959)[19] proposes simple granular degeneration, which he has been able to demonstrate in the rat.*

The bladder develops from the superior half of the primitive urogenital sinus, which is that portion above the opening of the mesonephric ducts. This portion of the urogenital sinus is the *vesicourethral* canal, and is responsible for the formation of the bladder and *primary urethra*. The portion of the urogenital sinus lying below the openings of the mesonephric ducts is the *urogenital sinus proper*. In the 21-mm embryo, a circular constriction appears between the orifices of the mesonephric ducts and the cephalad-migrating ureters. This constriction marks the border line between the bladder and urethra and represents the vesical neck (Fig. 5).

By the second month of development, the bladder has expanded into an epithelial sac with its apex tapering upward to the umbilicus, as the *urachus*. There is considerable controversy regarding the contribution of the allantois to the upper portion of the bladder. It seems reasonably established that the bladder base and primary urethra are derivatives of the cloaca, whereas the remainder of the bladder is developed from the allantois.[272, 555, 394, 8]

THE URETHRA

The urogenital sinus proper, that portion of the primitive urogenital sinus lying below the opening of the mesonephric ducts at Müller's tubercle, is further divided into two portions: a proximal, short one, lying directly below Müller's tubercle, and a distal, longer one, which

---

*Either of these hypotheses could account for the supramontane folds frequently seen in the normal prostatic urethra, and in some cases where they are excessively prominent could correspond to the valvular role ascribed to them by Young and Frontz (type II valves). Obstruction due to these folds is probably quite rare. Ectopic ureteral orifices lie at or above the verumontanum in the male and have not been described opening distal to the female urethral meatus.

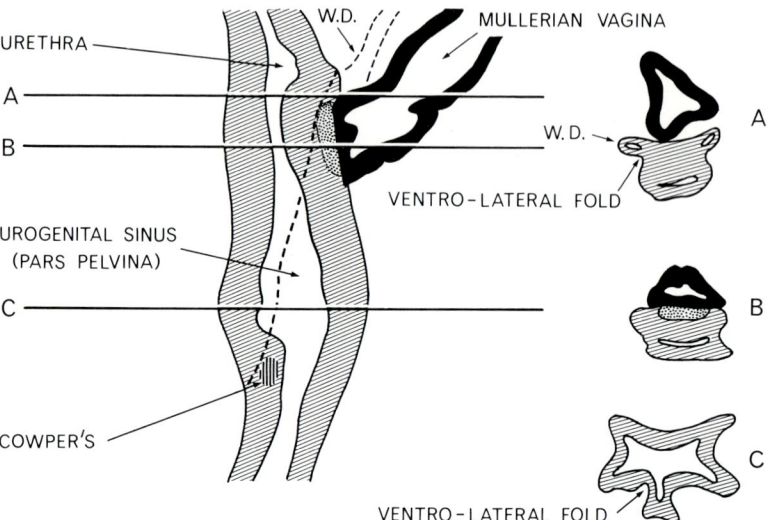

FIG. 6. Diagram to show site of the developing urogenital sinus (pars pelvina) contribution to the lower portion of the vagina in the 70-mm female sheep fetus; the ventrolateral folds (precursors of the anterior portion of the hymenal ring) are indicated by the heavy dotted line; the relations of the wolffian ducts and Cowper's gland anlage to this fold are shown in sagittal section (left) and horizontal section (A, B and C right). (Redrawn from Bulmer.[59])

develops in its walls longitudinal ridges (*Seitenwandleisten*), at the distal portions of which ultimately develop Cowper's and Bartholin's glands and duct systems (Fig. 6). Toward the proximal end of these ridges in the female, a horizontal ridge develops on the underside (dorsum) of the urogenital sinus, and pouches posteriorly and cephalad to join with the vaginal plate. This is the *Kaudelzapfen* of Politzer[407,348,58,59] or the "camera retrohimenal" of S. Gil Vernet. It is the precursor of the vagina. There is some evidence to indicate that the upper four-fifths of the vagina develops from the müllerian duct complex (Koff,[279] Felix,[147] Forsberg[155]), and that the lower fifth has its source in this distal portion of the urogenital sinus. Koff[279] postulated that the lower portion of the vagina arose by the growth of paired "sinovaginal bulbs" from the dorsal sinus wall. The fusion and subsequent cavitation of these initially solid epithelial outpouchings then form this vaginal segment.

The studies of Bulmer in the sheep[58,59] and the human,[60] while in essential agreement with the urogenital sinus origin of the vaginal epithelium as described by Vilas[510,511] and Koff,[279] led him to conclude that in the human the *entire* vaginal epithelium arose from these "dorsolateral wings" of urogenital sinus epithelium. Rather than finding that this unique type of sinus epithelium formed distinct bulbous structures—suggesting some type of symmetrical budding—Bulmer conceived the sinus epithelial invasion as a dorsolateral epithelial investment, cleft in the midline by the mesodermal projection of the fused müllerian ducts. J. Davies and Kusama[107a] in 1962 presented excellent evidence, in the human fetus, to confirm Bulmer's observations, and quite flatly state that the human vagina is entirely of urogenital sinus origin. Jones and Scott[258] similarly pointed out that in the studies of the prostatic utricle in the human by Vilas (1933)[511] and in the mouse by Raynaud (1942)[427] the "prostatic utricle" was constituted from an outgrowth of the urogenital sinus which extended *under* the müllerian ducts. These authors consider that the "prostatic utricle" is more closely analogous to the vagina than to the uterus.

In this view, the border line between that portion of the urogenital sinus contributing to the formation of the primary (sphincteric) urethra in both sexes can be considered the junction of the proximal and distal segments of the urogenital sinus proper, rather than the formerly accepted level of the verumontanum, and the primary (sphincteric) urethra can be considered to have the same length in both the male and the female (Kjellberg, Ericsson and Rudhe[272]).

Bulmer,[60] in the 120-mm human fetus, found that the sinus upgrowth of the urogenital portion of the vagina extended for a distance of approximately 1.6 mm. In the 140-mm female fetus, the lower end of the vagina communicates with the urogenital sinus by paired hymenal orifices, separated from each other by a small median mesodermal septum. The hymenal folds bounding the outer ventral margins of these paired orifices represent the dorsal margins of the *urethrovaginal folds* of the earlier stages. The mesodermal septum between the two hymenal orifices differs in origin from the remainder of the hymen. This septum is projected forward, probably by the downgrowth of the vagina and, thus, divides the space between the dorsal margins of the urethrovaginal folds (Koff[279]).

The original oblique urethrovaginal folds assume a more transverse position in the female to form the ventral half of the hymen. In the male the cranial vestiges of the urethrovaginal fold appear to remain

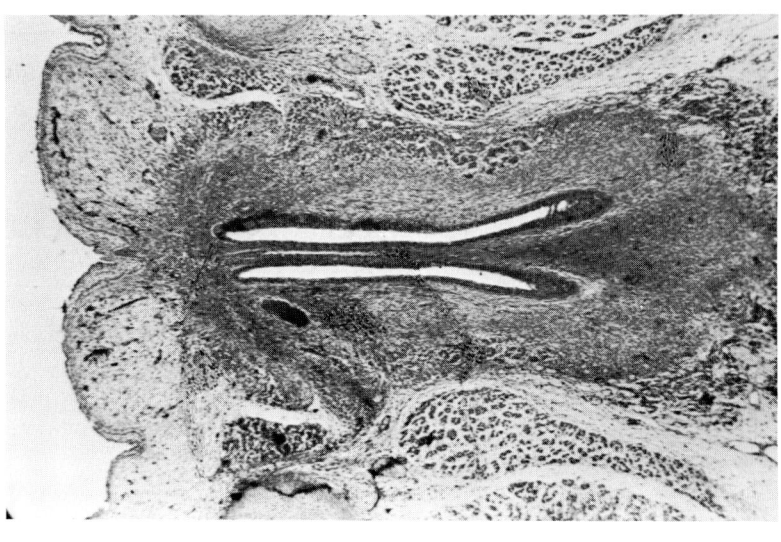
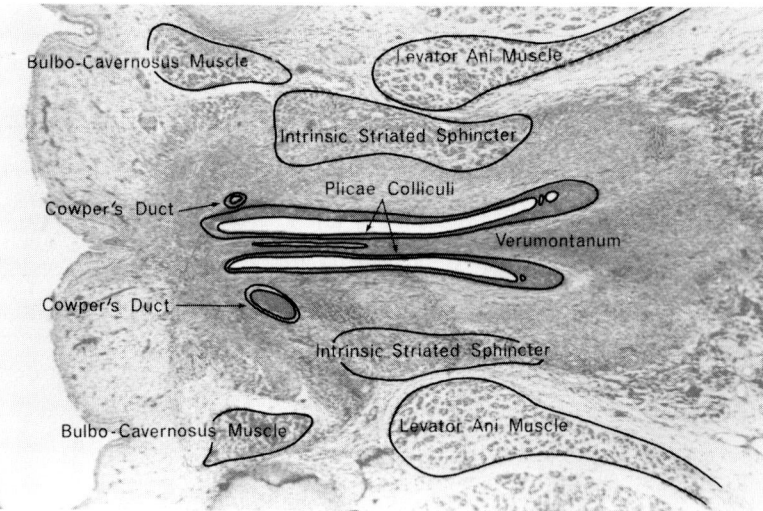

FIG. 7. *A*, 55-mm male embryo. Frontal section of the developing inframontane urethra. The bifid plicae colliculi (crista urethralis) extending into the future bulbomembranous urethra. Note the position of Cowper's ducts *proximal* to their distal limits. The plicae in the male are the analogues of the anterior portion of the hymenal ring in the female. Original magnification X40.

as the plicae colliculi with their distal ends buried in the walls of the bulbomembranous urethra and their proximal extremities terminating beneath the verumontanum. Their dorsal, and usually parallel, disposition along the *floor* of the inframontane urethra results from the lateral migration of the originally ventrally inserted urethrovaginal folds, aided to some extent by the lateral growth and fusion of the bulbous and cavernous portions of the male urethra from the phallic portion of the urogenital sinus. A similar mechanism probably accounts for the final posterolateral, and closely adjacent, positioning of Cowper's glands between the two layers of the urogenital diaphragm (Fig. 7A).

The great enlargement of the lower end of the vagina in later stages results in an extension of its area of contact with the sinus, particularly in the lateral and caudal aspects. In its posterior half, the hymen is formed by a buckling inward (or pleating) of the urogenital sinus wall.[279] The hymenal ring thus has two mechanisms of origin and consists of a plate of dense connective tissue lined above and below by the differentiated sinus epithelium which occupies the upper part of the sinus. In the male the cavernous urethra develops from the distal phallic portion of the open urogenital sinus proper by infolding of the edges of the urogenital groove on the undersurface of the phallus as far as the coronal sulcus (Fig. 7B). The glandular urethra is formed by canalization of an ectodermal cord of cells which unites with the cavernous urethra proximally and the tip of the glans penis distally. In the female, the phallic portion of the urogenital sinus remains open as the vestibule. The urethral meatus in the female is closely analogous to the point of the junction between the membranous and bulbous urethra in the male.

Anatomical Relations

The urinary bladder is a smooth-muscle walled, hollow viscus with a loosely attached *transitional cell mucosa*. The fibroelastic net of smooth muscle comprising the detrusor continues without interruption as the musculature of the urethra. The mucosa, except in the region of the trigone, rests upon an equally mobile tunica propria.

The arterial supply to the bladder is derived from three main sources: (1) *the superior vesical artery,* which provides the greatest territorial supply in that it branches over the anterolateral surfaces,

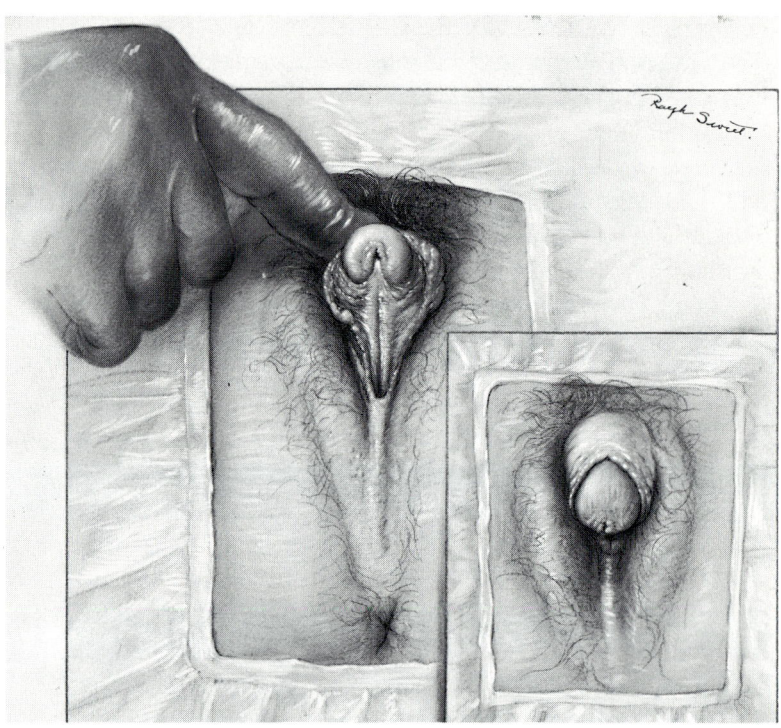

FIG. 7. *B*, Drawing depicting the anomalous development of the phallic portion of the urogenital sinus in intersexuality. The urogenital membrane has closed the pelvic portion of the urogenital sinus. The phallic portion has failed to close. The common urogenital sinus orifice in this case is just slightly distal to the urethral orifice.

(2) *the vesiculodeferential artery*, which supplies the posterior base of the bladder, the vas deferens and seminal vesicles, and (3) *the inferior vesical artery*, which supplies the anterior portion of the vesical neck and detrusor above it, as well as the prostate and seminal vesicle. These all arise from the internal iliac or its major branches. The inferior vesical artery is the most variable and arises from the internal pudendal or its branches in 60 percent of the specimens examined by Braithwaite[48] (Fig. 8). The venous return does not parallel the arterial supply, but drains into the extensive plexus of Santorini, prevesically and laterally. It is eventually returned to the inferior vena cava by the hypogastric veins.

The position and shape of the bladder within the pelvis vary with the volume of its contents. Its most usual configuration when observed from within the pelvis is that of an irregular ellipse with a flattened or slightly concave vertex. Only with distention to capacity does it assume the globular shape usually conceptually ascribed to it (Fig. 9).

Although an extraperitoneal organ surrounded on its anterior and lateral surfaces by the loose areolar tissue of the space of Retzius and its lateral perivesical recesses, the superior surface of the bladder is covered with firmly adherent peritoneum for approximately one-third the area of its vertex. Posteriorly, the supratrigonal surface is again free of dense connections so that, upon penetrating the peritoneal reflection of the posterior cul-de-sac, the extraperitoneal areolar tissue isolating the rectum in the male and the uterus in the female can be easily pushed aside in the midline to expose the posterior wall of the bladder.

Laterally and caudally, the ureters, inferior vesical vessels, and the pelvic portion of the hypograstic plexus can be identified. Below the level of the interureteric ridge in the male, the posterior base of

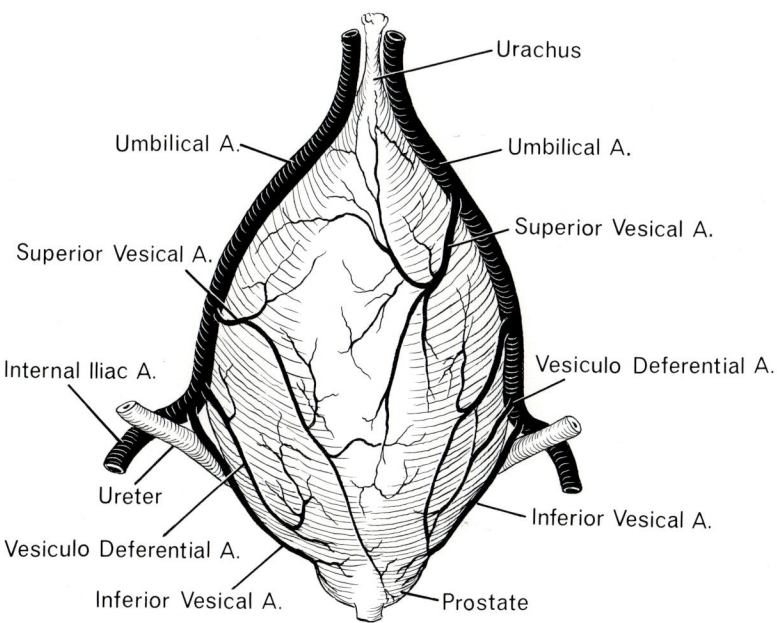

FIG. 8. The arterial blood supply to the anterior surface of the infant bladder. (After Braithwaite.[48])

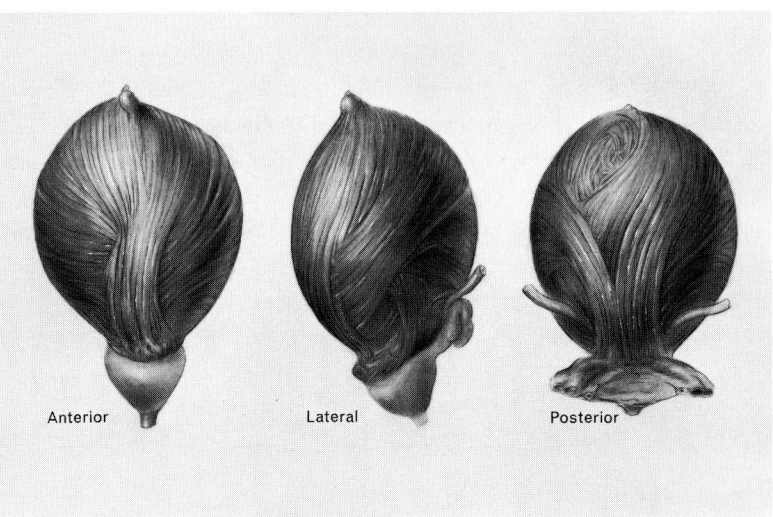

Anterior Lateral Posterior

FIG. 9. Drawings made from a gross dissection of the bladder in a 6-year-old male child, showing the usual muscle bundle distribution. There was considerable variation in the pattern noted in five other specimens from children under the age of 5 years. The variations were most frequent in the upper two-thirds of the bladders. The distribution of the longitudinal, oblique and looped musculature of the lower thirds was remarkably constant.

the bladder is firmly united with the seminal vesicles and prostate and separated from the rectum by the tough rectovesical layers of Denonvilliers' fascia. In the female, the subtrigonal vesical musculature is intimately adherent to the anterior vaginal wall. Passing distally to the urethral meatus, there is a progressively firmer alliance of the vaginal wall with the musculature of the vesical neck and urethra.

The position of the urinary bladder is maintained primarily by its urethral and vascular connections. In the male, the membranous urethra is firmly grasped by the superior and inferior fibrous layers of the urogenital diaphragm which is, in turn, anchored solidly to the periosteum of the inferior pubic rami. The bladder and prostatic urethra can neither descend below this level nor rise above the limits imposed on the muscular urethral column by its attachments to the triangular ligament. Only with the shearing of the membranous urethra, or disruption of the pubic rami, can the bladder float up into the pelvis.

In the female, the urogenital diaphragm is a less solidly constructed set of layers. The same principles of fixation apply, however, except that the female urogenital diaphragm is more subject to prolonged stress and strains of disruptive force which tend, with age and childbearing, to interfere with its functional integrity. The fixation of the female urethra to the anterior vaginal wall commits it to share in all the difficulties of fixation to which the latter is heir.

Of less importance than the urethral connections of the bladder is its support by the pubovesical bundles. In the male these are frequently called the puboprostatic ligaments, and in the female the pubovaginal ligaments. The inferior vesical vessels and ureters are inadvertent tethers for the upper border of the trigone and posterior bladder base. The markings on the peritoneal surface of the bladder, the urachus and the remnants of the hypogastric arteries (or false ligaments of the bladder) are little more than fibrous festoons in their normally obliterated states. They have no supporting function.

The striated muscles of the perineum, including the levator ani and deep transverse perineal muscles, provide only secondary fixation for the bladder insofar as they are attached to the fascial structures surrounding the urethra.

Musculature of the Bladder and Sphincteric Urethra

Gross Anatomy

The detrusor muscle, rather than being regarded as an inexplicable smooth-muscle meshwork with an outer longitudinal and an inner circular layer, should be regarded as a meticulously coordinated system of smooth-muscle fiber bundles continuous with the sphincteric urethral musculature. Uhlenhuth pointed this out clearly in 1953.[506] In the careful dissections of Uhlenhuth and Hunter, illustrated by William Loechel, it is possible to trace individual fiber bundles from a longitudinal arrangement on the anterior and posterior surfaces of the bladder, through progressive decussations to ever deeper levels within the detrusor. Here the bundles assume first a circular arrangement, subsequently an internal longitudinal orientation of the anterior wall of the bladder, and ultimately a stellate reticular set of terminations at the vertex.

In the literature, there are numerous descriptions of specific fiber bundles of the bladder and vesical neck. Portions or groups of smooth-muscle fiber bundles have been frequently redescribed and selectively emphasized with specific functions attributed to them (Bro-Rasmussen, et al.,[49] H. H. Young and Wesson,[565] Hutch,[240] Manley,[330] Tanagho and Smith,[487] Hunter[238]). Woodburne,[553] in his studies of the musculature of the base of the bladder and urethra, emphasized the fixation of the anterior longitudinal layer to the pubis via the pubovesical bundles. Lapides[299] correlated the anatomy with a major event in the act of micturition—the shortening of the sphincteric urethra based on the continuity of the longitudinal smooth-muscle fiber bundles of the detrusor with those of the urethra. Hutch has demonstrated that "urethral funneling" noted cineradiographically is due to elevation of the muscular "base plate" during voiding.[243,244,245]

Today a clear understanding of the anatomy of the bladder and urethral musculature must rest heavily on the definitive histotopographic description of S. Gil Vernet. The studies of Hutch,[243,240] Uhlenhuth, Hunter and Loechel,[506] Woodburne[553,554,555] and Lapides[301,297,299,298] are indispensible to the balanced consideration of vesical structure. There are, however, still many controversial areas and unresolved conflicts of anatomical structure with function.

The basic concept is that the detrusor muscle is composed of an organized set of interlacing smooth-muscle fiber bundles which are continuous, anatomically and physiologically, with the smooth-muscle bundles in the sphincteric urethra of both male and female. Further, the smooth-muscle bundles of the urethra are intimately associated with the special ("intrinsic") striated muscle surrounding the sphincteric urethra, and their functions are neurologically synergistic (Bors,[33] Rolnick,[440] S. Gil Vernet[173,175]). The bladder and sphincteric urethra of the male and the entire female urethra to its meatus within the vestibule can be regarded as continuous muscular cylinders (Marberger[335]) (Fig. 10).

Descriptions and an attempt at resolution of the anatomy as defined separately by Uhlenhuth, Hunter, S. Gil Vernet, Hutch, and Woodburne are necessary here. Although certain structural points are extremely important, of necessity the discussion must be more abbreviated than these authors deserve.

Hunter[238] points out that "the outer longitudinal musculature of

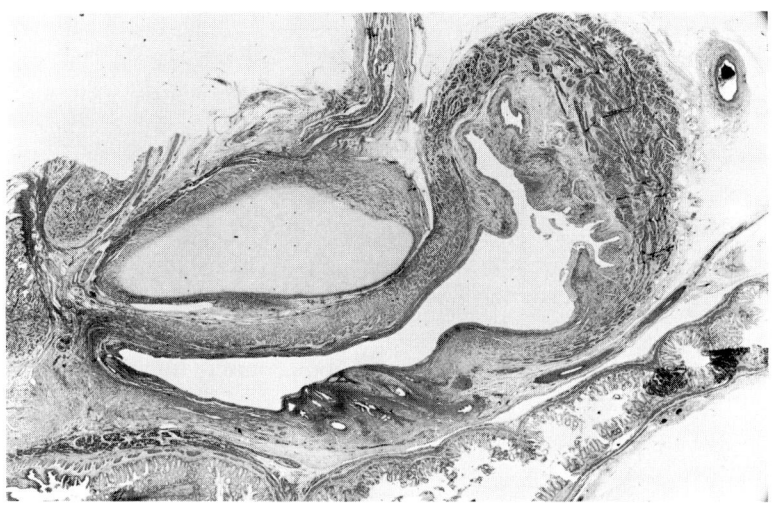
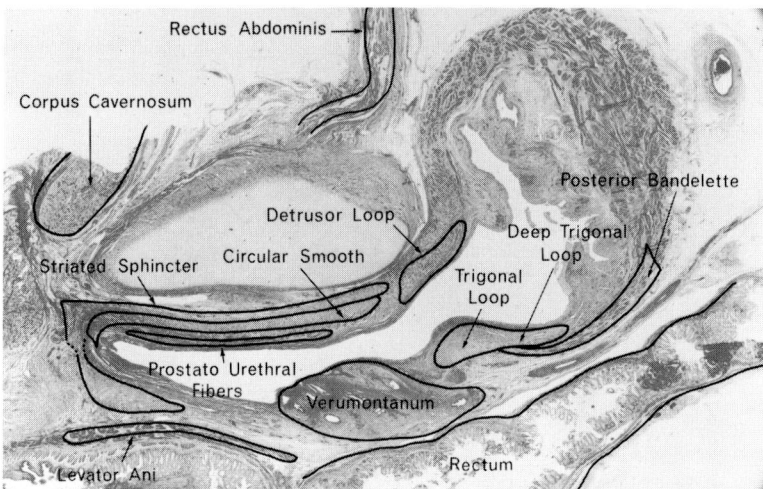

FIG. 10. Midline sagittal section of 170-mm (5-month) human fetus to show continuity of the musculature of the detrusor with that of the sphincteric urethra.

the bladder is arranged in two layers, a dorsal layer and a ventral layer. Both layers are stratified into a superficial group and a deep group . . . the ventral layer is approximately one half the thickness of the dorsal group." He found that the bundles of the dorsal layer could be traced from the dorsal portion of the *internal sphincter*, and that some of the fiber bundles penetrated into the middle lobe of the prostate gland in the male.*

Hunter was able to follow the ventral layer from (1) the *pubic bone*, by way of the pubovesical bundles, (2) the *ventrum* of the *internal sphincter,* and (3) a *musculotendinous* band attached to the periphery of the base of the prostate gland in the male.

Hunter, Uhlenhuth and Woodburne all agree with the Kalischer concept of muscular attachments of the detrusor to the periosteal fibrous tissue beneath the pubic bone (pubovesical bundles). S. Gil Vernet contends that these are only minor and insignificant continuations of the anterior longitudinal smooth-muscle bundles into the pubovesical bundles, and observed that the anterior longitudinal fibers inserted into the anterior portion of the internal sphincter (superficial detrusor loop) and the musculotendinous band surrounding the prostate (superior prostatic aponeurosis) (Fig. 11).

*It would seem that "cranial lobe of the prostate" is a better term.

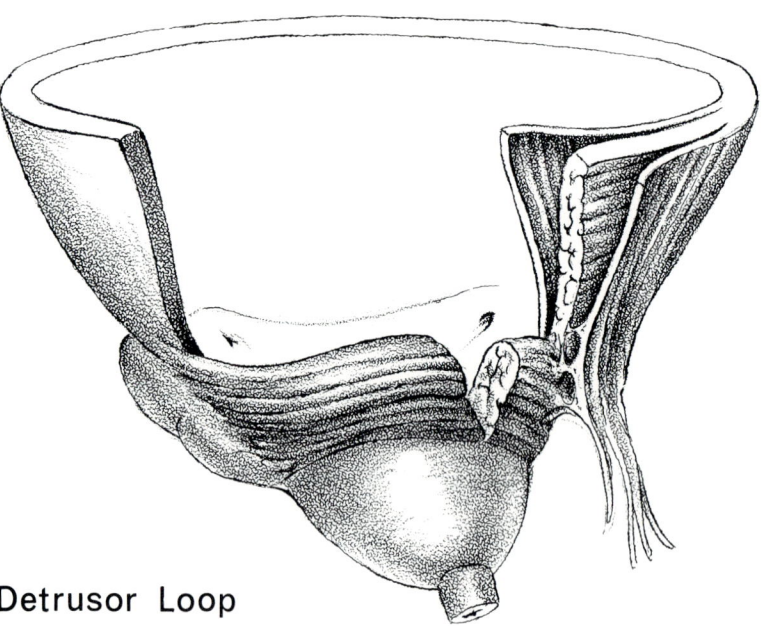

Detrusor Loop

FIG. 11. Drawing of a gross dissection specimen from a 6-year-old male child to show the relations of the detrusor loop with the longitudinal and circular musculature in the lower one-third of the bladder.

There are differences between the number and manner of decussations between the superficial longitudinal groups and the deep longitudinal groups, the latter eventually dividing into small circular bundles intermingling with the circular bundles from the superficial layers to become indistinguishable from them. The innermost longitudinal layer of the bladder anteriorly is a continuation of the original superficial and deep ventral longitudinal layers which have become circular and subsequently aligned themselves with the long axis of the bladder. At the apex of the bladder, the inner longitudinal muscles form a stellate mass. Basally, they form a plexus of fibers which is situated along the lateral and ventral periphery of the internal orifice of the urethra, and gives rise to the thick layer of lateral and ventral inner longitudinal musculature of the urethra.[506] These are the anterior and lateral vesicocervical fibers described by Versari.[509]

The deep posterolateral fiber bundles have a different distribution from that of the superficial longitudinal anterior and posterior fibers. Uhlenhuth stressed the course of these deeper fiber bundles on the posterolateral bladder wall and traced them in a circular course both anteriorly and posteriorly about the bladder neck. This is the most difficult concept in the study of the bladder musculature. He also pointed out their contributions to the extrinsic longitudinal musculature of the ureters. Uhlenhuth, while describing a ventral loop of muscle fibers coursing about the vesical neck, as well as a parallel group, regards the *trigonal loop* as a complete ring in itself and, in effect, the "internal sphincter."

Hutch and Shopfner[244] regard the combination of these looped bundles of the vesical neck as forming a "base plate" demonstrable on cineradiography. In Hutch's view, the most cephalad of the ventral vesical neck loops is properly an extension of the deep subtrigonal transverse fibers, while the caudal portion of the ventral loop is a continuation of the posterolateral fiber bands of the detrusor.

In the classic European view, there are again these two opposing arcs comprising the internal sphincter mechanism. These are the two *horseshoes* ("Hufeisen," "demilunes") which can be visualized to intersect obliquely, in their separate but complementary planes, to form the "internal sphincter." It is generally thought that these tissue components of the vesical neck are pulled aside by the active contraction of *all* of the longitudinal smooth-muscle bundles extending along the urethra to permit micturition. Woodburne denies the exist-

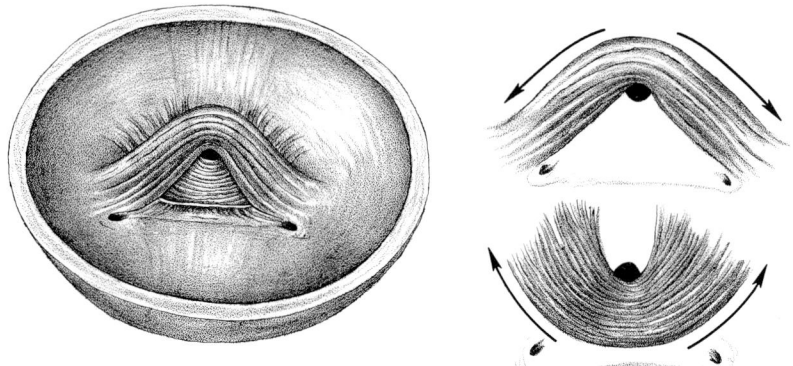

FIG. 12. Diagrammatic view from within the bladder showing the arcuate musculature of the vesical neck (detrusor and trigonal loops) intersecting in oblique but mutually complementary planes. This complex, together with the post-trigonal transverse bundle, forms the "base plate" (Hutch). Surgically and radiologically it represents the "internal sphincter" or vesical neck. Superficial trigonal muscle has been excised to demonstrate the muscle bundle distribution.

ence of a discrete annular internal sphincter and also doubts the existence of arcuate closing of the vesical neck. From his studies, he postulates that these bundles arch *past* and *away* from, rather than *around*, the vesical neck. In Woodburne's view, elastic tissues of the vesical neck and spongy vascular spaces in the tunica propria act as the passive internal sphincter.

S. Gil Vernet describes the internal sphincter mechanism as a functional one composed of superficial and deep detrusor loops and the trigonal loop functioning together (Fig. 12). This relationship can be well demonstrated histotopographically. It is certainly not an annular ring, nor do these bundles arch away from the vesical neck. It seems impossible to deny these powerful detrusor fiber bundles a major role as a functional internal sphincter on clinical, surgical, and anatomical grounds.

Histotopographic Anatomy of the
Urinary Bladder
(as described by S. Gil Vernet)

I. Muscle Bundles of the Detrusor
   A. Anterior Group
      1. Anterior Longitudinal Bundle

      2. Lateral Bundles (paired)
      3. Inner Anterior Longitudinal Bundle
   B. Posterior Group
      1. Posterior Longitudinal Bundle (bandelette)
      2. Posterolateral Longitudinal Bundles (paired)
         a. "Interior" Fascicles
         b. "Exterior" Fascicles

II. Muscle Bundles of the Vesical Neck
   A. Trigonal Loop
   B. Detrusor Loop
      1. Superficial (Heiss)
      2. Deep (Gil Vernet)
   C. Transverse Precervical Arc
   D. Pubovesical Bundles
   E. Superficial Trigonal Muscle
   F. Post-trigonal Transverse Bundle
   G. Interureteric Ridge (Mercier's bar)

III. Muscle Bundles of the Sphincteric Urethra
   A. Vesicocervical Fibers
      1. Anterior
      2. Lateral
      3. Posterior (superficial trigonal muscle)
   B. Vesicoprostatourethral Fibers
   C. Sub-sphincteric Arc Fibers
   D. Prostatourethral Fibers
      1. Anterolateral
      2. Posterior
   E. Vesicourethral Fibers (female)
   F. Cervicourethral Fibers (female)

IV. Intrinsic Striated Muscle of the Sphincteric Urethra
   A. Superior
   B. Middle
   C. Inferior

V. Circular Smooth Muscle of the Urethra
   A. Internal (genital) Sphincter
   B. External (inframontane and membranous) Sphincter
   C. Sphincter of Albarran

Histotopographic Anatomy

In serial sections of the bladder and sphincteric urethra in infants, fetuses, and adults, S. Gil Vernet established a smooth-muscle bundle structure which is continuous from the musculature of the detrusor to its most distal insertions in the intrinsic striated portions of the sphincter and the mucosa of the membranous urethra.

Rather than to consider the musculature of the bladder as "arising" at the vesical neck, as Uhlenhuth and Hunter described it, it is more accurate to reverse the concept, and to trace the musculature of the bladder as it *continues into* the sphincteric urethra.

THE SMOOTH-MUSCLE BUNDLES OF THE URINARY BLADDER

The detrusor bundles of smooth muscle in the lower third of the bladder can be shown histotopographically to form demonstrable groupings. These are most conveniently considered as *anterior* and *posterior* groups.

The anterior group includes:

1. *Anterior Longitudinal Bundle.* This is the outer longitudinal bundle coursing from the vertex of the bladder to insert at the vesical neck into the transverse precervical arc. Other fibers continue to form a point of fixation in the retropubic connective tissue. Woodburne has called this insertion the "pubovesical bundle." This connection was originally pointed out by Kalischer and corresponds in surgical terminology to the pubovesical ligaments.
2. *Transverse Precervical Arc.* This arises from the lateral longitudinal bundles of the detrusor, receives fibers of the anterior-longitudinal bundle, and abuts closely (but is superficial and ventral to) the detrusor loops. Its configuration is in the form of a short arc with its concavity directed posteriorly. From this confluence of fibers, longitudinal fibers descend distally to blend with the pubovesical bundle, the vesicocervical and cervicourethral fibers.
3. *Paired Lateral Bundles.* These have their origin in the vertex of the bladder, contribute to the transverse precervical arc anteriorly and to the retrosymphysial vesicourethral system (pubovesical bundle, vesicourethral and cervicourethral fibers).
4. *Inner Anterior Longitudinal Bundle.* This is a group of slender fibers immediately beneath the tunica propria which interdigitate with each other at the vesical neck to form a slender muscular web of *plexiform*

fibers. Their distal continuations become the vesicocervical fibers (Versari) and eventually terminate in the ventral urethral mucosa at a point opposite the verumontanum (Fig. 13).

The posterior group includes:

1. *Posterior Longitudinal Bundle (bandelette).* This is the heaviest and most prominent muscle bundle of the entire detrusor system. It inserts broadly into the deep transverse trigonal muscle. Other fibers are anchored in the midline to the cranial prostate in the male and to the cranial portion of the urethrovaginal septum in the female. The more lateral fibers give rise to anterior vesicoprostatourethral fibers, which course around the vesical neck in company with the "externa" portions of the posterolateral-longitudinal bundles. These latter eventually blend with the retropubic vesicourethral system and some of them interdigitate with the superior division of the intrinsic striated sphincter.
2. *Paired Posterolateral Longitudinal Bundles.* These are responsible for the formation not only of the all-important detrusor loop and its divisions but also for the "interna" portions, which are deflected medially to become continuous with the heavy transverse post-trigonal bundle fibers.

The posterolateral bundles can be separated somewhat arbitrarily into two groups: (1) *medial* ("interna" of Gil Vernet) to the ureteral penetration of the bladder, and (2) *lateral* to it ("externa" of Gil Vernet).

Circular detrusor fibers are seen between the inner and outer longitudinal bundles, but lie well above the vesical neck and are not essential to this further description.

THE SMOOTH-MUSCLE BUNDLES OF THE VESICAL NECK

The *trigonal loop* is a bundle of slender transverse arcuate fibers, the terminal ends of which are anchored in the lateral portions of the transverse precervical arc and detrusor loops anterolaterally. Ventral to this and immediately beneath the mucosa of the trigone is the superficial trigonal muscle which has a longitudinal distribution and runs from the interureteric ridge to the verumontanum, where it inserts into the mucosa of the urethra.

Beneath and slightly cranial to the trigonal loop is the deep transverse trigonal muscle arising from the posterolateral longitudinal bundles. This is composed of thicker fibers, and receives the insertions

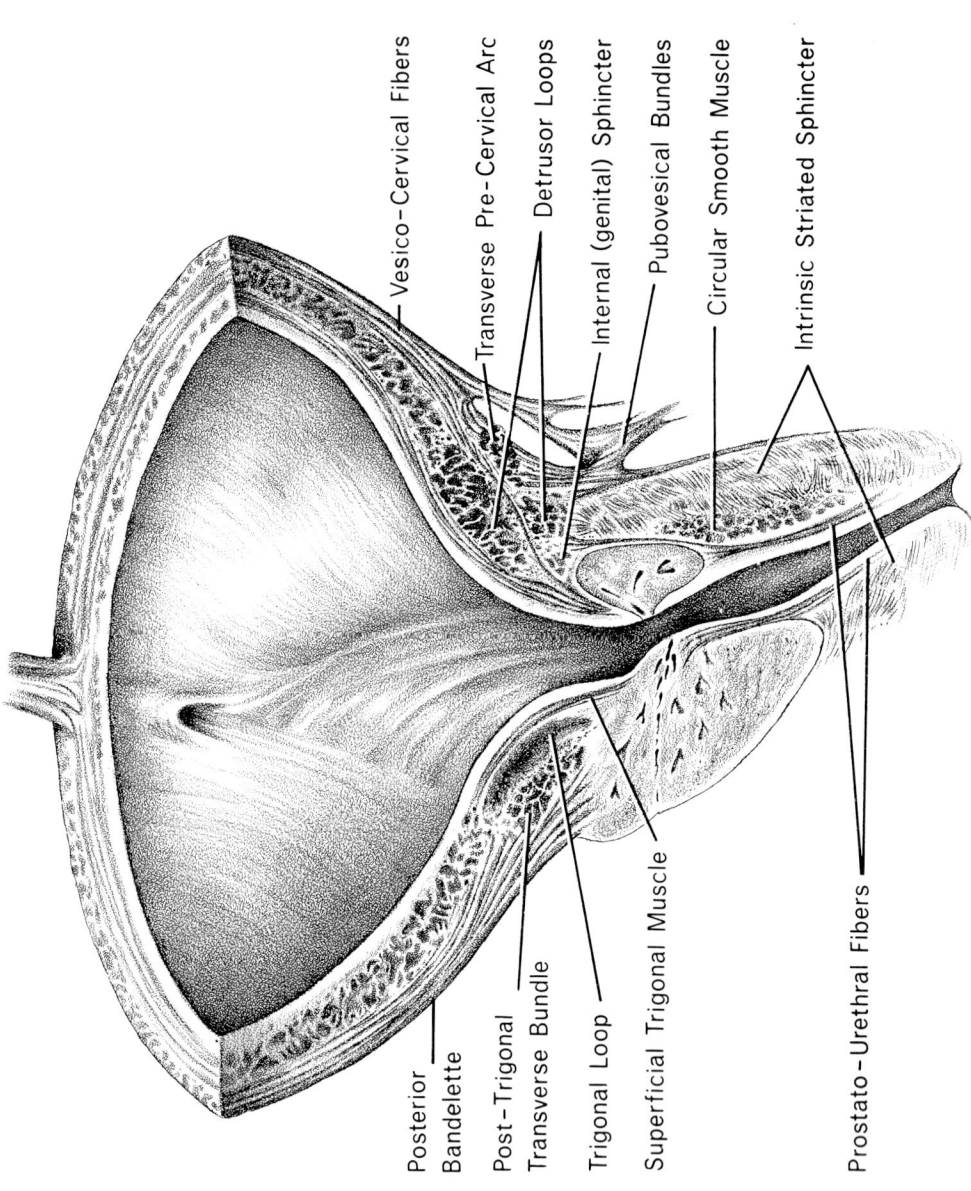

FIG. 13. Drawing to show the course and insertions of the principal muscle bundles of the sphincteric urethra.

of the posterior longitudinal bundle (bandelette) in the form of microscopic tendinous attachments at right angles to the directions of its fiber bundles. These are the "petits tendons" or "tendoncillos" of Gil Vernet, and were also noted by Wesson in 1920,[531] Rolnick and Arnheim[440] and Gireaux.[177]

The *detrusor loop* can be divided into two parallel coursing loops. These arise from the heavy posterolateral longitudinal bundles of the detrusor after they have split to give off the previously described deep transverse trigonal muscle. The detrusor loop, instead of running posterior to the internal urethral orifice, becomes splayed out into two separate bights, lying anterior (ventral) to the vesical neck. The most distal of these and the most deeply imbedded in the urethrovesical junction is the *profunda* (Gil Vernet), while the shorter and more cephalad is the *superficial* (Heiss). These partially split loops lie respectively caudal and cephalad to the transverse precervical arc, but *deep* to it. The detrusor loop represents the classic anterior horseshoe, with its concavity directed backward and upward (dorsocephalad). This probably represents one of the bundles which Woodburne described as arching away from the vesical neck.* The profunda portion, particularly, contributes a number of longitudinal fibers to the anterior segment of the muscular urethral cylinder (Fig. 14).

THE MUSCULATURE OF THE SPHINCTERIC URETHRA

The musculature of the urethra is composed most importantly of longitudinal smooth-muscle bundles continuous with the major detrusor bundles, which come to form a smooth-muscle cylinder around the urethra. Although partially surrounded by the prostate in the male, the urethra has its own muscular integrity.

The *vesicocervical fibers* are the immediately submucosal longitudinal slender bundles, which can be conveniently divided into anterior, lateral and posterior groups. The anterior vesicocervical fibers arise for the most part from the inner (anterior) longitudinal bundle of the detrusor by way of an intermediate anastomotic bed of *plexiform* fibers. These longitudinal fibers course through the vesical neck and terminate in the mucosa of the urethra at the level of the verumontanum. There are supplementary fibers of this group coming from

---

*The deep transverse trigonal muscle may be another.

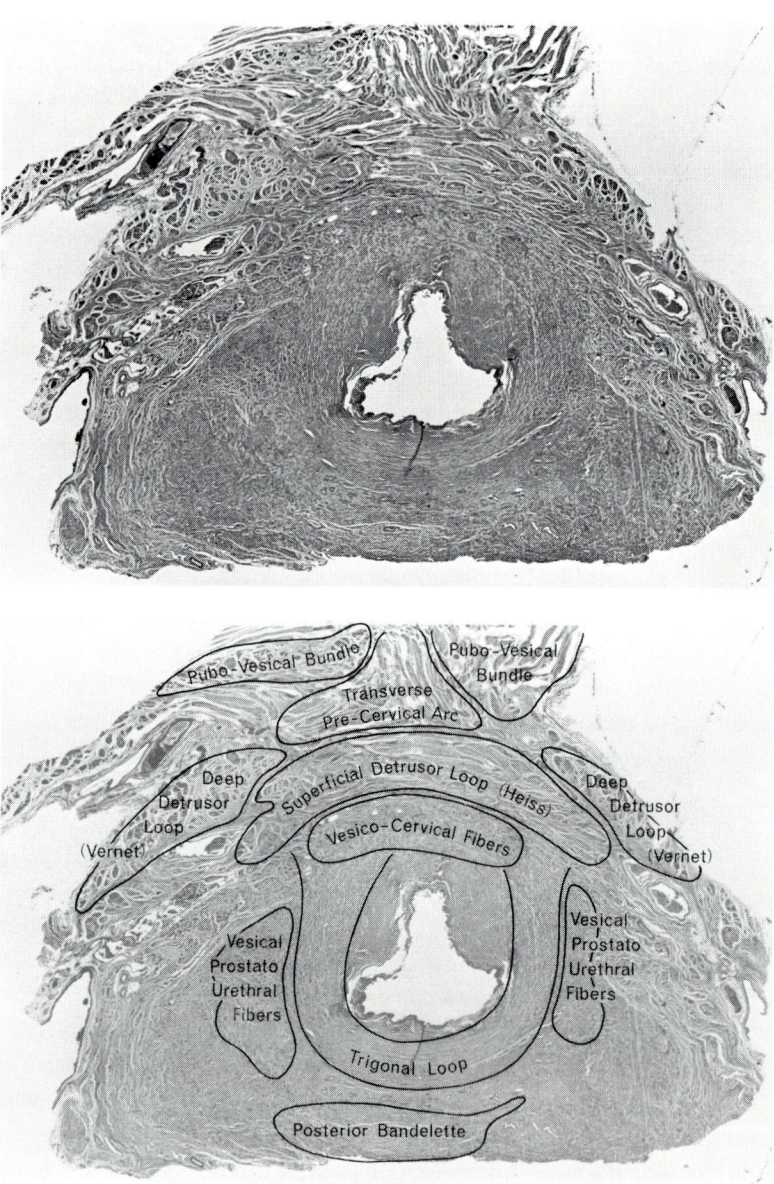

FIG. 14. Horizontal section from the vesical neck of a 2-year-old human male showing distribution of the sphincteric urethral musculature. Level is the insertion of the posterior bandelette into cranial prostate. The trigonal loop is prominent. Superficial trigonal muscle fibers cannot be identified in this section. Photomicrograph above and tissue map below. Verhoeff-van Gieson stain. Original magnification X15.

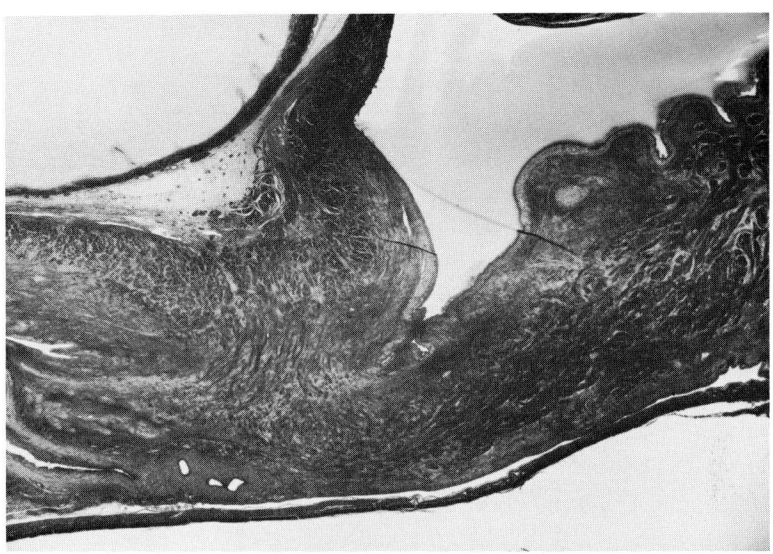
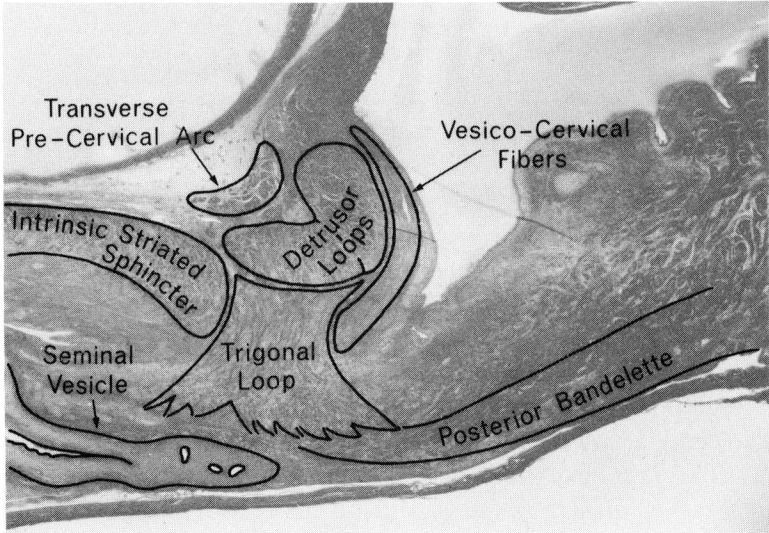

FIG. 15. Sagittal section of the vesical neck in a 430-gm (5-month) male fetus showing distribution of the trigonal and detrusor loops. Mallory azan stain. Original magnification X25.

the detrusor loop (deep), as well as from the anterior longitudinal bundle (Fig. 15).

The rather sparse *lateral vesicocervical fibers* arise in a manner similar to the anterior ones, in part from the plexiform fibers but also from the penetrating fibers of the lateral longitudinal bundles of the detrusor. The insertions into the urethral mucosa are the same as that described for the anterior vesicocervical fibers.

The *posterior vesicocervical fibers* are primarily the fibers of the superficial trigonal muscle;[531, 330, 565, 487] they appear in serial sections actually to arise from the tunica propria (or mucosa) of the trigone itself, while other fibers arising from the trigonal loop join with them to pass through the vesical neck posteriorly to insert into the mucosa of the verumontanum. There is still much controversy as to whether or not the superficial trigonal fibers are continuations of the intrinsic longitudinal musculature of the ureters. Bell[18] proposed that only the lateral borders of the superficial trigonal muscle arose in this manner and inserted into the submucosa of the verumontanum. Others[324, 565, 486, 240] attributed this distribution to the entire trigone. Tanagho and Smith believe that the entire superficial trigonal muscle is a continuation of the longitudinal ureteral musculature.[487]

Woodburne,[555] S. Gil Vernet[171] and Stephens and Lenaghan[474] find no continuity with the intrinsic longitudinal musculature of the ureter. This musculature, they believe, can be demonstrated to terminate in the mucosa of the trigone at the ureterovesical orifice, except for a continuation of the intrinsic ureteral musculature to form the interureteric ridge (Mercier's bar). The exact origin of these slender, and frequently absent, fibers is still in doubt (Fig. 16).

The *vesicoprostatourethral fibers* are so named because they do not have the limited course of the vesicocervical fibers. These fibers arise from the posterior-longitudinal bundle and run longitudinally along the sphincteric urethra outside the vesicocervical fibers. Other parallel fibers of this group run peripheral to the intrinsic striated external sphincter. These fibers do not terminate in the mucosa, but continue the entire length of the sphincteric urethra.

To this group of fibers belong the *sub-sphincteric arc fibers*, which form a recurving, open-ended, flattened ellipse with the closed portion of the arc located posteriorly beneath the internal (genital) sphincter. The distal limbs are in contact with the striated muscle of the membranous urethra.

The *prostatourethral fibers* are longitudinal, submucosal smooth-muscle bundles pursuing the same plane which the vesicocervical fibers abandoned upon their insertion into the mucosa of the urethra at the level of the verumontanum. The prostatourethral fibers arise as two

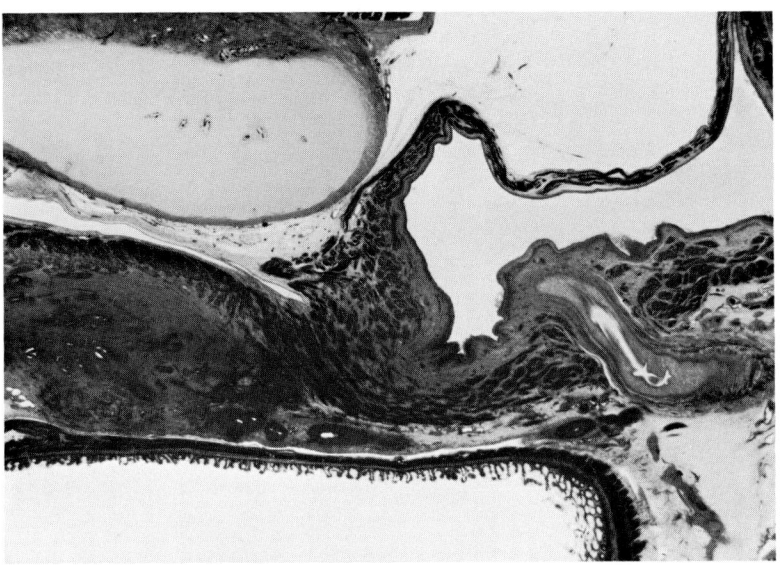
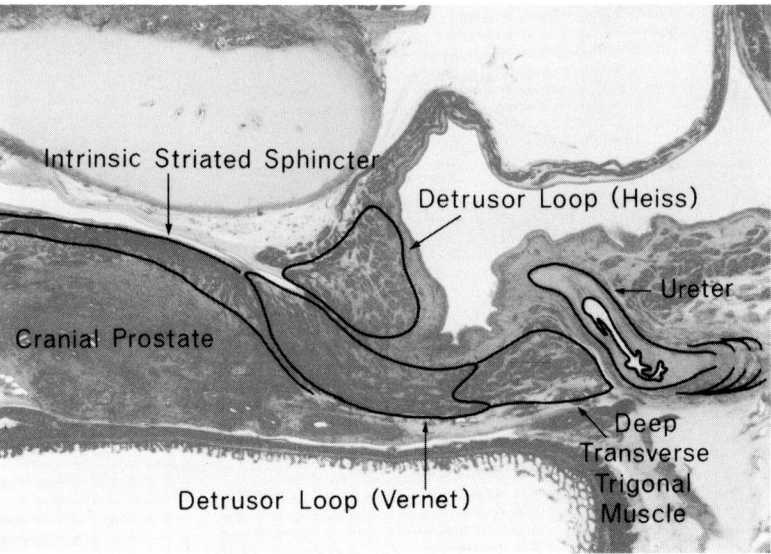

FIG. 16. Parasagittal section through ureterovesical junction showing relation of ureteral and trigonal musculature. 430-gm male fetus. Original magnification X15.

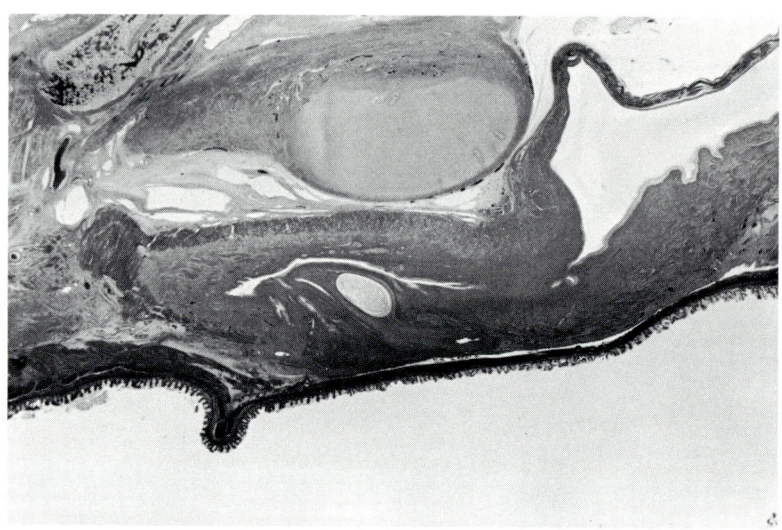

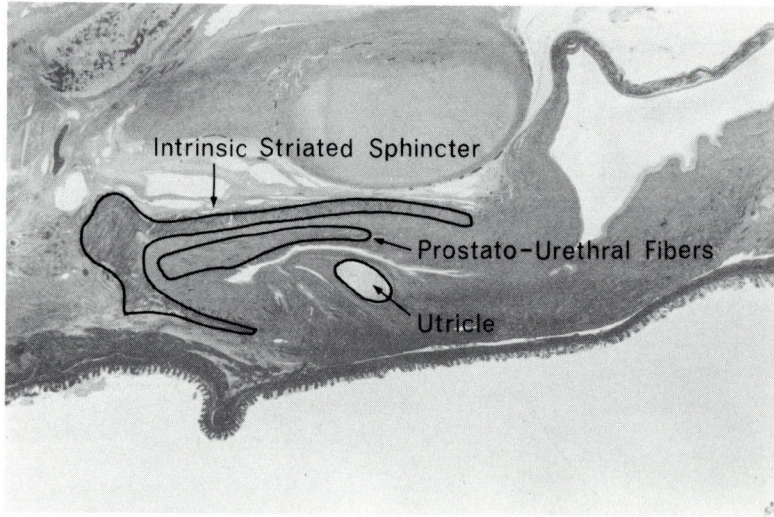

FIG. 17. Parasagittal section showing distribution of the intrinsic striated sphincter and prostatourethral fibers. 430-gm male fetus. Magnification X15.

major groups: (1) the anterolateral and (2) the posterior. The anterolateral arise from stroma of the anterolateral portion of the caudal prostate (Fig. 17).

In the first part of their longitudinal course toward their insertion into the mucosa of the inframontane and membranous urethra, some fibers turn medially to join with opposite similar fibers above the anterior wall of the urethra opposite the verumontanum. Other fibers of the posterior vesicocervical system continue laterally around the verumontanum to join the posterior prostatourethral fibers.

The posterior fibers, which are not only smooth muscle but densely interlaced with elastic fibers, arise in a discrete bundle from the verumontanum, *beneath* the caudal wall of the utricle, to contribute to the substance of the inframontane crista urethralis (plicae colliculi). These delicate myoelastic fibers fan out somewhat laterally along the floor of the inframontane urethra as they progress to their insertion in the submucosal layers of the bulbomembranous urethra.

THE INTRINSIC STRIATED MUSCULATURE
OF THE SPHINCTERIC URETHRA

It has long been known that the striated muscle surrounding the urethra was not limited to a particular area such as the membranous urethra in the male or the distal urethra in the female (Kalischer,[259] Marion,[339] Albarran[1, 224]). During transurethral resection striated muscle is frequently fround in specimens "removed from the vesical neck."[34] McCrea[365] noted striated muscle in the trigone. Slips of striated muscle can indeed be identified on the posterolateral portions of the deep transverse trigonal muscle (Manley,[330] S. Gil Vernet,[171] Haines[201]). There is some controversy about the innervation of this striated muscle. Most observers hold firmly that it is innervated as other voluntary muscle by somatic nerves, specifically the muscular branch of perineal nerve arising from the deep branch of the pudendal nerve. Other workers in animal and human studies have found no connections of the pudendal nerve with these particular striated muscle fibers, with the exception of the sheep.[174, 175, 548, 549]

The intrinsic striated muscle surrounding the urethra in the male forms a complete ring only in the membranous urethra. Here, it lies outside the circular smooth muscle which, in turn, lies peripheral to the longitudinal periurethral smooth-muscle fibers in the prostato-urethral system. The urethral striated muscle here has no connections with the levator ani fibers except for a slender midline connection known surgically as the "rectourethralis muscle," nor is there a relation to the striated muscle surrounding Cowper's glands. It is, however,

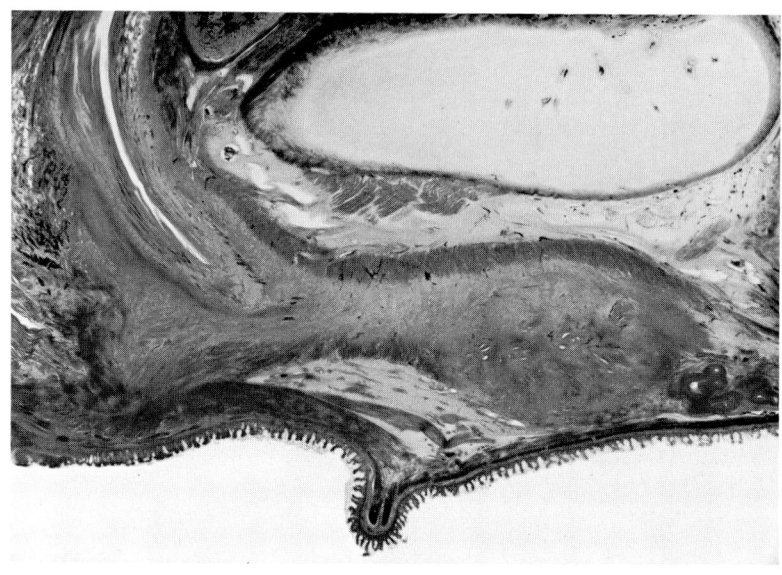
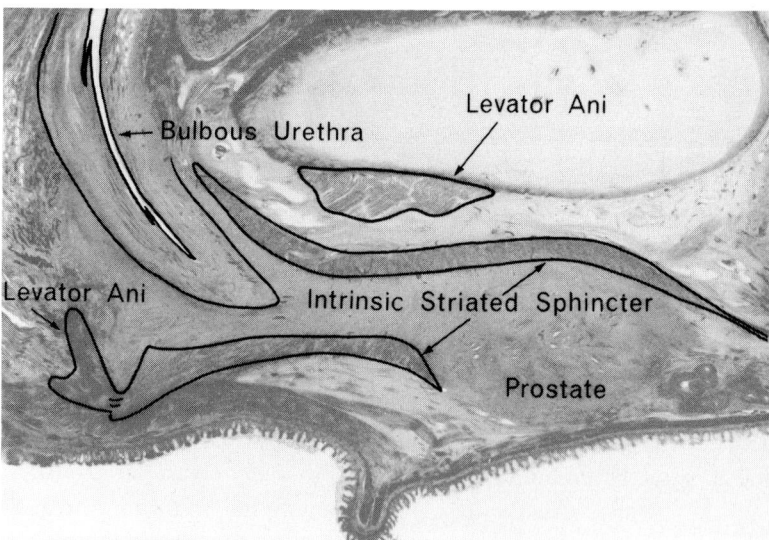

FIG. 18. Parasagittal section of sphincteric urethra showing distribution of intrinsic striated sphincter and its sole connection ("rectourethralis muscle") with fibers of the levator ani.

related by tendinous or appositional connections to the longitudinal (vesicoprostatourethral fibers) and circular smooth muscle of the inframontane urethra (Fig. 18).

In reviewing serial sections approaching the vesical neck (from caudal to cranial) in male specimens, the striated muscle is seen progressively to lose the posterior half of its circular fibers so that it assumes a saddle-like position on the ventral aspect of the sphincteric urethra. This middle portion of the striated urogenital sphincter can be considered to be the *prostatic portion*, for it arches around the anterior (ventral) surface of the prostate. The fibers of the inferior (caudal) portion of this arc in the region of the inframontane urethra are arranged in an oblique plane which can be imagined to run from the apex of the triangular ligament toward the anterior anal verge. As sections progress cranially, the fibers change direction slightly so that the medial fibers in the region of the verumontanum have a transverse, ventral, arcuate distribution about the urethra. Above this level, at the vesical neck, the superior fibers assume a progressively oblique aspect, paralleling an imaginary plane from the vesical neck anteriorly toward the bases of the seminal vesicles posteriorly; and the uppermost fibers continue posterolaterally to interdigitate with the lateral smooth muscle of the post-trigonal transverse bundle and "interna" portion of the posterolateral longitudinal bundle well above the vesical neck (Figs. 19A, B).

The female urethra presents the same appearance except for the fact that there is an even less complete circular striated muscular ring, and this only in the middle third of the urethra. Distal to this, the striated muscle is inserted laterally into the vaginal septum and continues to the urethral meatus in this ventral arcuate relationship. In the region of the vesical neck it again, as in the male, forms only a half circle anteriorly and has similar deep trigonal connections.

CIRCULAR SMOOTH MUSCLE OF THE MEMBRANOUS URETHRA

This layer consists of anterior arcuate smooth-muscle bundles lying immediately beneath the striated muscle of the inframontane and membranous urethra. These fibers arise from the stroma of the caudal lobe of the prostate and form an anterior arc embracing the anterior longitudinal prostatourethral fibers. In the membranous urethra these

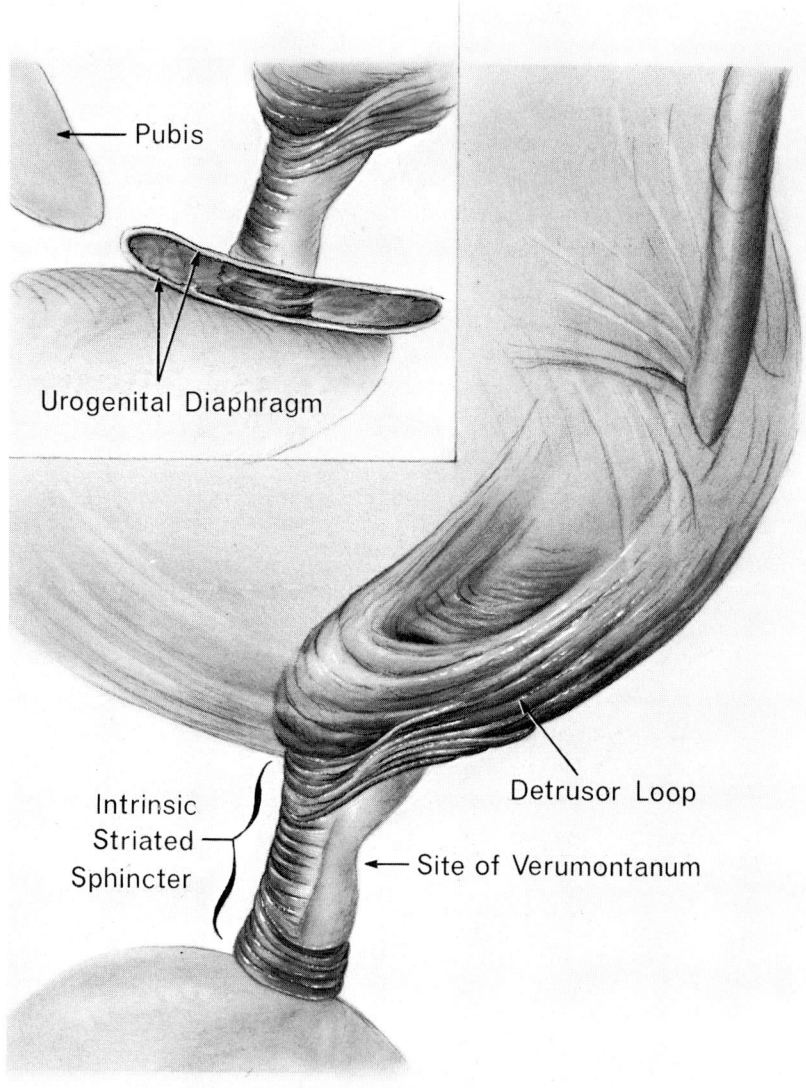

FIG. 19. *A*, Diagram to show the distribution of the intrinsic striated sphincter. Note that it is not limited to the space between the two layers of the urogenital diaphragm. It extends the entire length of the sphincteric urethra ventrally, and has insertions into the smooth muscle of the detrusor loop dorsolaterally.

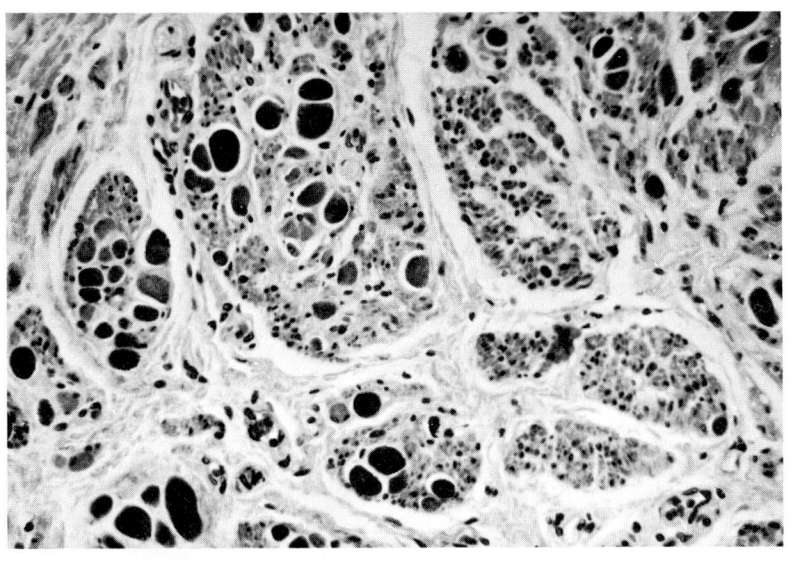
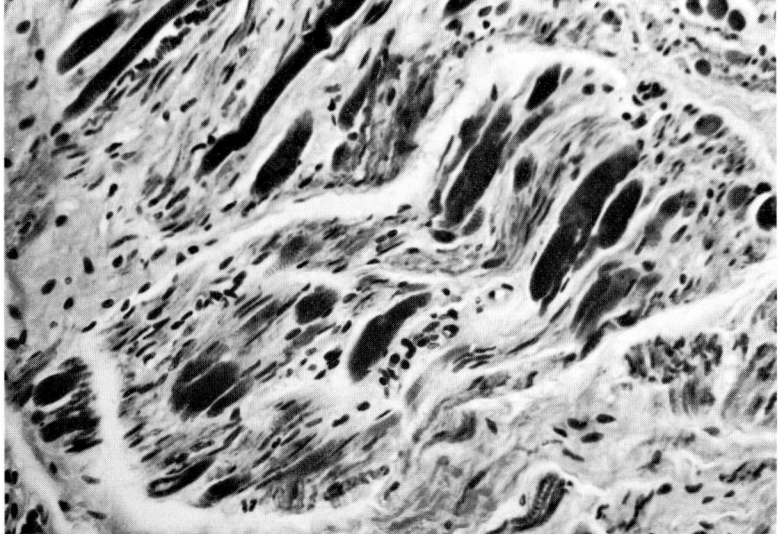

FIG. 19. *B*, Attachments of the most cranial fibers of the intrinsic striated sphincter to posterolateral longitudinal bundles of the detrusor in the deep trigonal musculature. Intermingled striated and smooth-muscle cells surrounded by a common perimysium suggest an unique type of mutual force transference, as yet unexplained. Muscle bundles are sectioned transversely (above) and obliquely (below). Striated fibers are densely stained. Apposed smooth-muscle cells are somewhat paler. Masson trichrome stain. Original magnification X250.

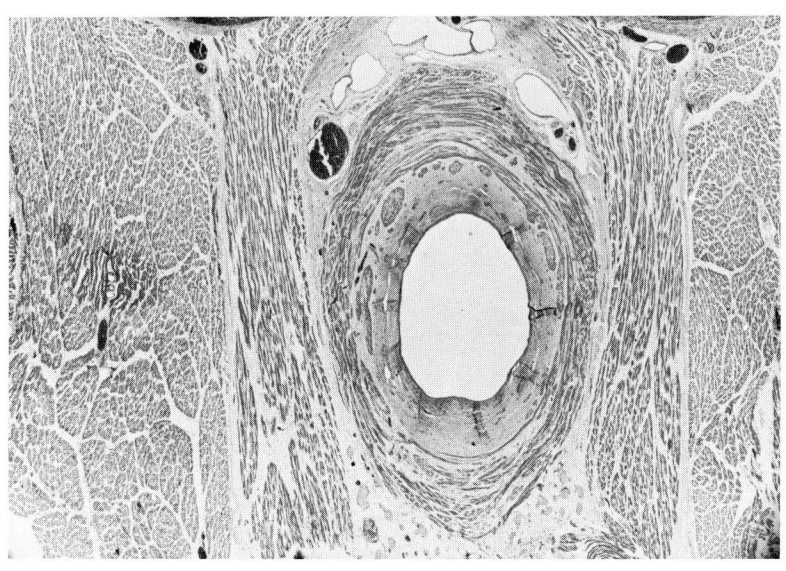
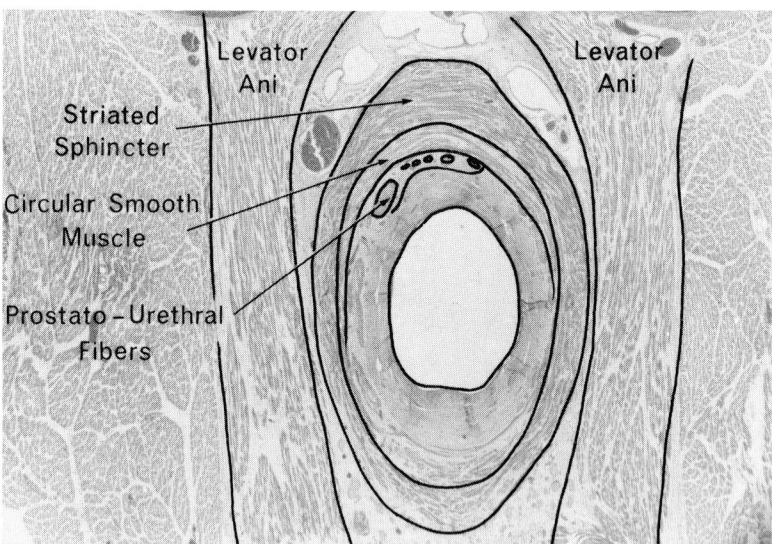

FIG. 20. Horizontal section of membranous urethra in 150-mm (5-month) human male fetus. There are complete rings of inner smooth muscle and outer intrinsic striated muscle. Note the lack of any continuity between the striated muscle of the levator muscles and the intrinsic striated musculature of the urethral sphincter. Section stained with Luxol fast-blue-Holmes' silver. Note the nerve bundles in the adventitia in each of the four quadrants. There is only a single ganglion at lower left. Original magnification X40.

fibers form a complete ring, but in the inframontane urethra only an anterior arc (Fig. 20).

The combination of the striated-muscle and the smooth-muscle elements, both circular and longitudinal, and Pennington's elastic dorsal submucosal arc investing them, comprise the clinical "external sphincter" portion of the sphincteric urethra.

CIRCULAR SMOOTH MUSCLE OF THE URETHRA

Distal to the sphincter of Albarran, which lies in the bulbous urethra just proximal to the openings of Cowper's ducts, there is no submucosal smooth muscle. The sphincter of Albarran is a definite, but slender, submucosal ring of smooth muscle lying 0.5 cm distal to the inferior margin of the membranous urethra (the internal meatus of Guyon). It is 10 to 20 μ thick in the 150-mm fetus and shows no connections with the longitudinal prostatourethral fibers. It is indeed a circular island of smooth muscle, which probably does not properly belong to the sphincteric urethra inasmuch as it has no detrusor connections. Its postulated function as a sphincter may be preventing reflux of Cowper's secretions. It serves no known purpose in normal urination.

CIRCULAR SMOOTH MUSCLE OF THE VESICAL NECK

On serial section, a circular, smooth-muscle ring, canted slightly forward immediately below the most distal extremity of the vesical neck, can be demonstrated. This is separate and distinct from the detrusor and trigonal loops, and has been designated the "internal sphincter" (S. Gil Vernet). *Internal sphincter* has become a confusing term, although anatomically accurate; it is perhaps wiser, in view of its relatively unimpressive histotopographic and probable functional significance, to consider it simply as circular smooth muscle of the vesical neck or internal "genital" sphincter.

Its fibers, viewed in a sagittal plane, are limited above by the detrusor loop, immediately beneath the most superior portion of the prostate, and sandwiched between the longitudinal vesicocervical fibers below and the tranverse precervical arc above. This ring is absent in the female urethra.* It is difficult to separate it completely from

*It has not been possible in my material to identify either the internal "genital" sphincter or the sub-sphincteric arc, although they are clearly demonstrable in the sections of Professor S. Gil Vernet.

the intimately related fibers of the detrusor loop (profunda). Its posterior fibers lie above and closely related to the loop of the subsphincteric arc, which is part of the vesicoprostatourethral system.

THE VESICOURETHRAL MUSCULATURE IN THE FEMALE

The adult female urethra is embryologically analogous to the supramontane urethra in the male. Its muscular structure, however, is not. Main differences occur in the distribution of the intrinsic striated and anterior longitudinal smooth-muscle bundles. The muscle bundle structure of the female bladder and the sphincteric urethra is comparable, however, to that described in the male. All of the female fiber bundles are more delicate, and in some cases show a less organized pattern, than those of the male. There are important differences, however. There is only a poorly developed retrosymphysial system in the female, and the fibers of the anterior and lateral superficial longitudinal bundles establish a more tenuous communication with the periosteum of the pubis.

The transverse precervical arc is not so well defined as is that of the male, but it maintains the same connections with the detrusor and is the source, as well as the transmitter, of the anterior vesicourethral fibers which form the most prominent longitudinal musculature of the female urethra.

The *detrusor loops* and the *trigonal loop* are easily identified, and have the same distribution as in the male. The *posterior bundle* (bandelette) sends its small tendinous attachments into the *post-trigonal bundle*, while other fibers insert into the urethrovaginal septum (Fig. 21).

The longitudinal urethral fibers analogous to the *vesicoprostatourethral fibers*, although having a similar origin (i.e., from the posterior longitudinal bundle (bandelette)), are here called *vesicourethral fibers*. Their courses and connections with the intrinsic striated sphincter are the same as in the male.

The *anterior vesicocervical fibers* arise, in the female, from the inner anterior and lateral longitudinal bundles of the detrusor and course through the vesical neck in company with the *posterior vesciocervical (superficial trigonal muscle) fibers*. These insert, however, into the urethral mucosa at the junction of the upper and middle thirds of the urethra. This point represents the limit of the vesical neck in the female.

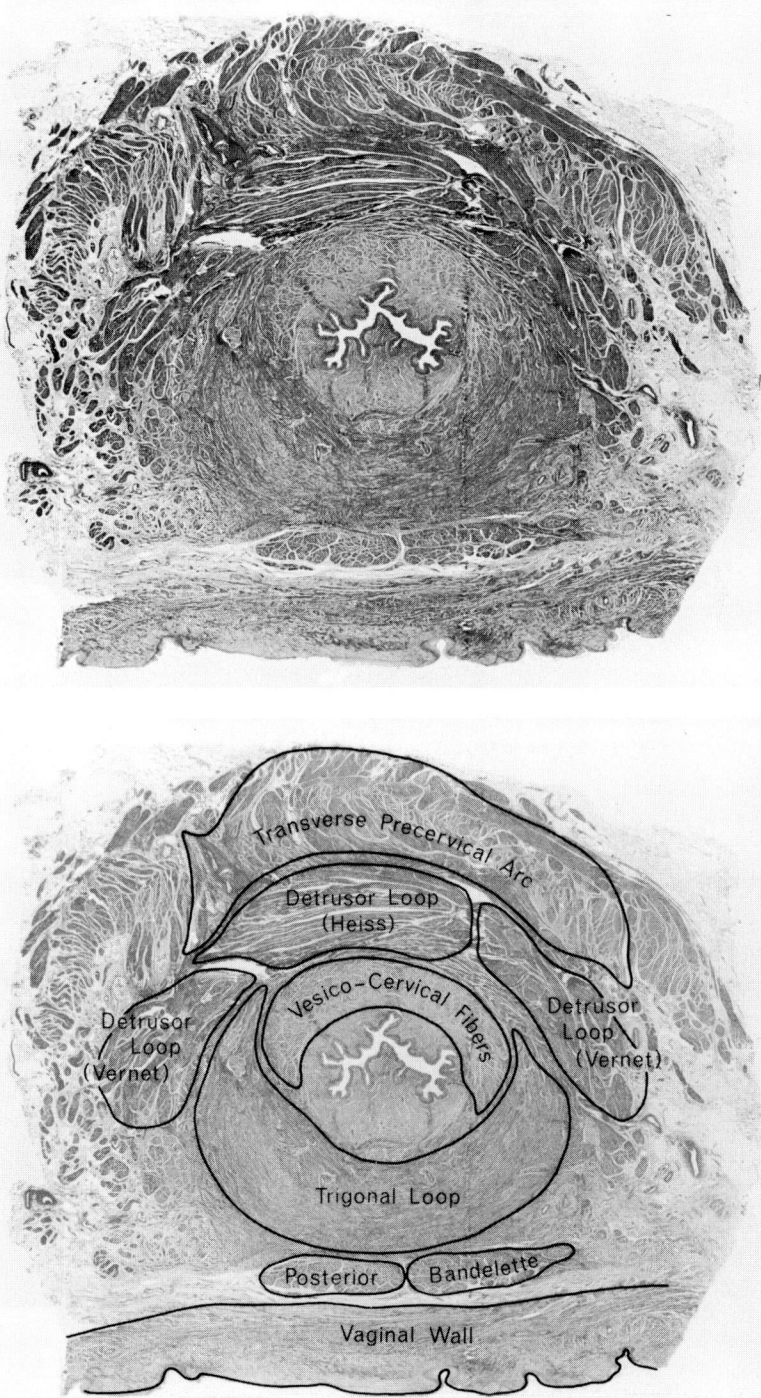

FIG. 21. Transverse section of the vesical neck in a 3-year-old girl. Note particularly the prominence of the anterior vesicocervical fibers and insertion of a portion of the posterior bandelette into the vesicovaginal septum.

The urethra below this contains longitudinal muscles of the cervicourethral system formed from the detrusor loop (deep). This longitudinal, submucosal musculature lies largely anterior and anterolaterally, and terminates just within the urethral meatus by appositional attachments to the intrinsic striated sphincter and insertions into the submucosa of the urethra. In the female there are no muscle bundles comparable to the *posterior prostatourethral fibers* (crista urethralis) in the male.

THE INNERVATION OF THE BLADDER AND SPHINCTERIC URETHRA

The bladder and sphincteric urethra are innervated by the autonomic nervous system via the hypogastric plexus. The fibers are of two types: sympathetic and parasympathetic. Of the two, the parasympathetic fibers can be said to be wholly responsible for both detrusor contraction and sphincteric function in the process of urination. There is good evidence to show that the striated perineal musculature (somatic innervation) is of only secondary and relatively minor importance in normal micturition.[298, 301, 141, 400]

Anatomically, the superior hypogastric plexus is located retroperitoneally at the level of the sacral promontory, and over the bifurcation of the aorta. Bifurcation of this plexus carries sympathetic fibers deep into the anatomical pelvis on either side, where they are joined by parasympathetic fibers (the *nervi erigentes*) originating in the second, third and fourth sacral segments of the spinal cord. These join to form the *inferior hypogastric plexus*. Thus joined, they form the *deep pelvic plexus*, which innervates the detrusor and the sphincteric urethra.

HISTOTOPOGRAPHY OF THE HYPOGASTRIC PLEXUS AND INTERNAL PUDENDAL NERVE

Main trunks from the inferior hypogastric plexus supply numerous branches to the detrusor; in descending past the vesical neck, they divide into two posterior cords, closely applied to the prostate and posterior urethra, and two anterior cords. The latter turn first horizontally at the vesicourethral junction and then longitudinally downward to the membranous urethra.

Two columns of nerves from the hypogastric plexus course along the posterolateral borders of the prostate and emanate from the perivesical ganglia. These show numerous gangliar interruptions and adventitial ganglia are most easily identified in the region of the vesical neck. Posterolaterally, ganglia decrease as these cords descend toward the membranous urethra, where they are eventually identified only as nerve bundles.

The prostate in horizontal section is roughly rectangular in shape, and these four cords occupy the anterolateral and posterolateral angles respectively.

In addition, a fifth cord is formed ventrally by small, horizontal anterior branches from the lateral main trunks. This descends anteriorly in the midline (Fig. 22).

The three anterior columns have few gangliar interruptions in the

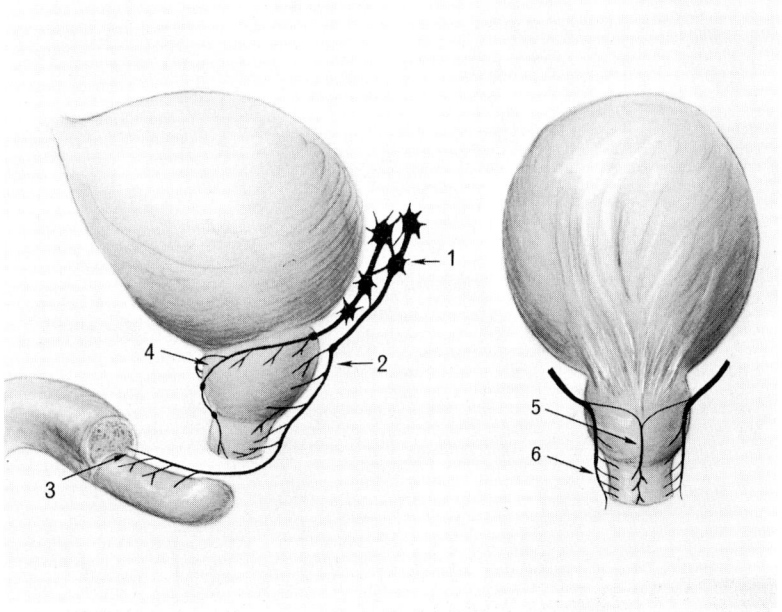

FIG. 22. Sketch of the histotopographic distribution of the five cords of the periurethral branches of the hypogastric plexus demonstrated by S. Gil Vernet. 1: Hypogastric plexus. 2: Posterior prolongation of the hypogastric plexus. 3: Nerves destined to supply the corpora cavernosae and corpus spongiosum. 4: Anterior prolongation of the hypogastric plexus. 5: Median anterior cord. 6: Anterolateral cord of hypogastric plexus. (Redrawn from S. Gil Vernet.[174])

perivesical plexus. The axons contain myelin, and terminations in motor end-plates among the muscle bundles of the intrinsic striated sphincter have been described.[174,175] There are numerous cross connections among all five of these longitudinal nerve columns, so that the prostate and membranous urethra are enmeshed in an autonomic collar. It is impossible at present to determine which fibers carry sympathetic, parasympathetic, sensory or motor impulses. The free anastomoses among these processes account for the minimal disturbance in function produced by ablation of parts of the hypogastric plexus.

All of the five vasculonervous cords terminate in the membranous urethra. In their descent they give up numerous branches to the prostatic as well as the inframontane urethra. The posterior cords also send branches into the corpora cavernosa and corpus spongiosum urethra.

Autonomic ganglia are most prominently distributed about the vesical neck and within the adjacent bladder wall (Fig. 23). These predominate in the superficial aspect of the muscle layers. The most promi-

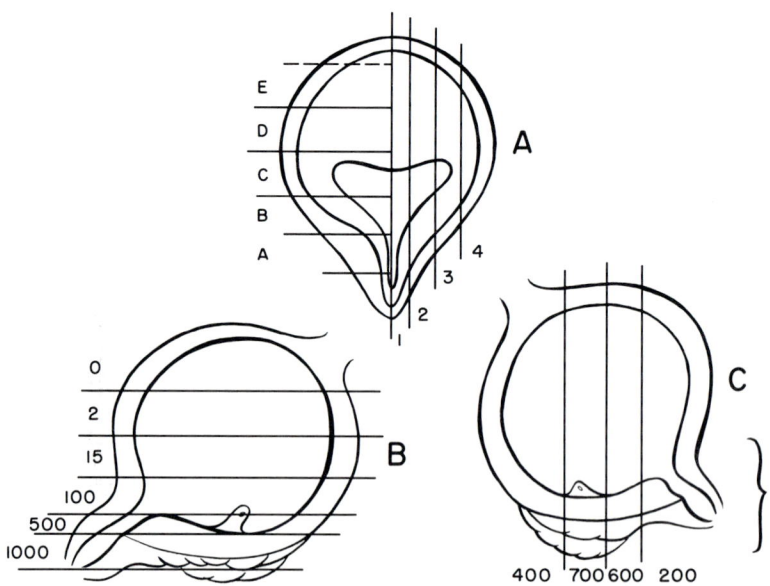

FIG. 23. Vesical ganglion distribution in lateral and transverse distribution in the newborn obtained by actual count in serial sections by Blanca Pavoli de Smith. (Courtesy of Dr. Smith.)

nent are in the adventitia, particularly posterolaterally in the region of the areolar tissues surrounding the base of the trigone, ureteral orifices, vas deferens and seminal vesicles.

As few as two ganglion cells or as many as a thousand may be noted within the individual ganglion. Where ganglion cells are found with ease in the superficial detrusor muscle, they are also found in appreciable numbers in the deeper muscle planes. Those deep within the muscle bundles commonly have fewer ganglion cells, on the order of two to ten per ganglion, as contrasted to the more densely populated adventitial ganglia.

Blanca Smith, in 1964,[463] in her studies of development of vesical ganglia, found some ganglion cells beneath the mucosa near the base of the bladder, but was unable to find these in the tunica propria of the fundus. She was able to count ganglia and identify preganglionic fibers, but had difficulty in identifying postganglionic fibers.

Vesical ganglia are considered to be a mixture of sympathetic and parasympathetic ganglionic fibers synapsing within the same ganglion. Evidence for this was obtained in cats by Kuntz, et al[287,288] by nerve root sectioning and subsequent examination of degenerated ganglia within the bladder wall. Kuntz and Mosely[287] showed that some ganglion cells degenerated and that others within an individual ganglion did not. They concluded from this that these were "mixed ganglia." They estimated that 40 percent of vesical ganglia were sympathetic, 40 percent parasympathetic, and 20 percent mixed, but that the distribution of sympathetic and parasympathetic ganglion cells in the trigone was approximately equal. Morphologically, it is difficult to differentiate cell types, and there is some confusion between simple maturation of the neuroblast from its apolar through bipolar and, subsequently, multipolar and neuroblast stages with ganglion cells which may have different (i.e., parasympathetic, sympathetic) structural and functional capacities (Dogiel,[118] Stöhr[476]) (Fig. 24).

Blanca Smith reported a "coming of age" of the primitive neurons during the fourth fetal month with a marked increase in Nissl substance and increasing organization of the dendritic processes, and noted that there was somewhat more precocious maturation of the ganglia in the adventitia than those in the muscularis.

The studies of El-Badawi and Schenk[131] confirm the mixed nature of the vesical ganglia in the dog, cat, rabbit and rat. In their studies they found three types of ganglion cells within the bladder

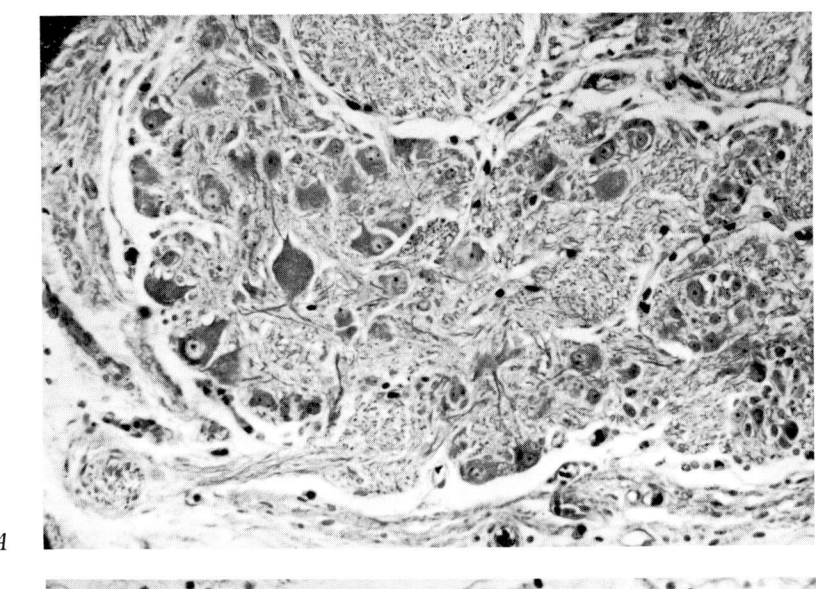

A

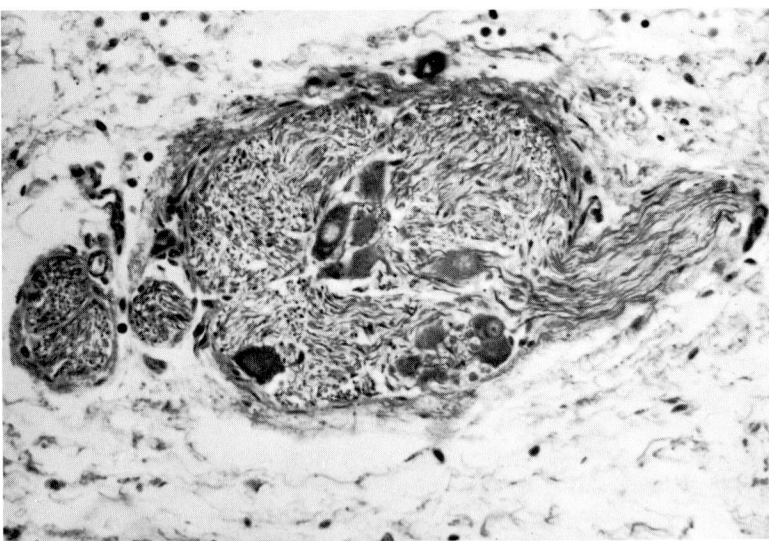

B

FIG. 24. Adventitial ganglia from the posterolateral bladder base in a 1300-gm premature male infant stained with Luxol fast-blue-Holmes' silver. Axons are densely black. There appear to be two populations of ganglion cells in *A*: large cells with abundant Nissl substance and multiple dendritic processes (left) and smaller, darker, less clearly structured cells at right. There is very little intermingling of the two cell types. A ganglion with emergent nerve is shown in *B*. All of the ganglion cells in this section are of the large type. Original magnification X250.

wall: (1) *Cholinergic cells* were the most frequently observed. They are cells rich in acetylcholinesterase (AChE) and associated only with cholinergic fibers, which ramified as postganglionic, presumably parasympathetic fibers. (2) *Adrenergic cells* were quite rare, containing only norepinephrine, which showed a diffuse bright green fluorescence. These gave rise to adrenergic postganglionic sympathetic fibers. (3) *Intermediate cell types* were commonly found and related to both cholinergic and adrenergic nerve fibers within the ganglia. Some stained heavily for AChE, others stained moderately or faintly for the enzyme and showed, as well, a diffuse faint or bright fluorescence and stippling with brightly fluorescent norepinephrine granules.

With differential stains for cholinergic and adrenergic cells taking advantage of the autofluorescence of norepinephrine and using an acetylcholinesterase stain, El-Badawi and Schenk determined that cholinergic and adrenergic ganglion cells existed in all layers of the bladder wall. They observed large cholinergic and adrenergic nerve trunks coursing in the adventitial coat of the bladder. Deep branches were found penetrating the muscularis and extending into the tunica propria. Also found were terminal cholinergic ramifications forming a neuroterminal plexus surrounding each smooth-muscle cell in the bladder wall. The adrenergic, postganglionic fibers formed networks of some complexity in the tunica propria and provided fine fibers to the epithelium. The adrenergic component of the perivascular plexus was the most prominent but there appeared to be some parasympathetic supply to blood vessels as well.

THE PUDENDAL NERVE

This somatic nerve originates from the ventral branches of S_2, S_3, S_4, and subsequently divides into two branches, the *dorsal nerve of the penis* and the *perineal nerve*. The dorsal nerve of the penis crosses the membranous urethra, but gives no branches to it.[174]

In the human, the perineal nerve divides into deep and superficial branches. The deep branch runs beneath the urogenital diaphragm, innervating the bulbocavernosus, ischiocavernosus muscles, the deep and superficial transverse perineal muscles, and the "sphincter urethrae membranacae" (Gray). Separate muscular branches, derived from the fourth sacral, innervate the levator ani muscles and the external anal sphincter. The superficial perineal nerve is distributed to the posterior scrotal skin in the male and labia majora of the female.

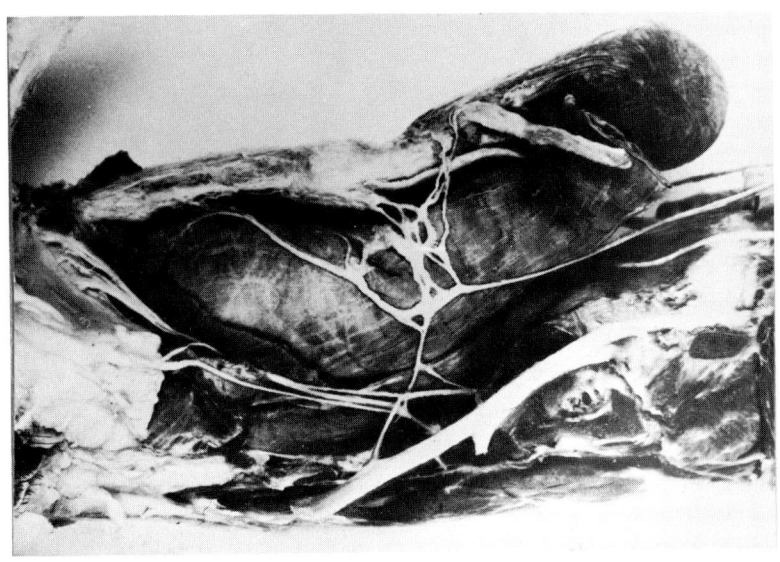

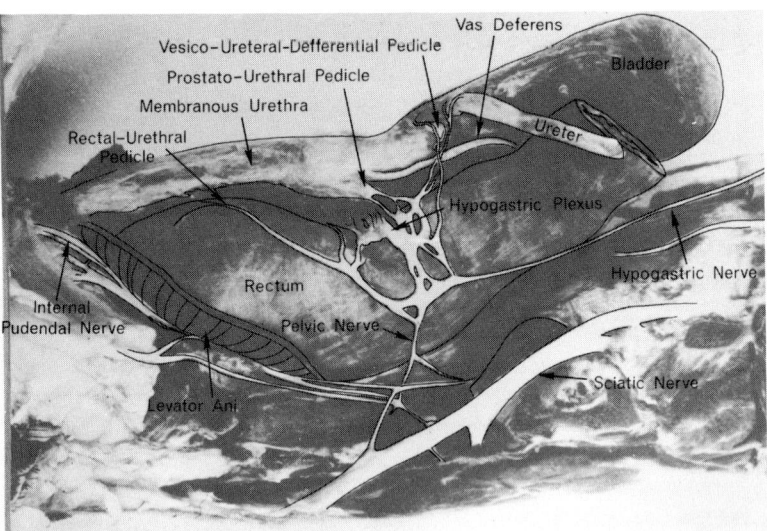

FIG. 25. Dissection of the hemipelvis of the dog (G. Winckler) of the autonomic and somatic nerves to the urethra, rectum and levator ani muscles. Note that there are no apparent connections of the pudendal nerve with the musculature of the sphincteric urethra. (Courtesy of Professor Winckler, Director of Institute of Anatomy, Faculty of Medicine, Lausanne.)

In the studies of S. Gil Vernet[174,175] in the human and Winckler[548,549] in the dog, no connections of the pudendal nerve or its branches with the intrinsic striated musculature of the sphincteric urethra could be demonstrated (Fig. 25).

Microscopic Anatomy

At the cellular level the bladder is composed of a 6- to 8-cell layer of transitional epithelium when the bladder is at rest. The connections among the epithelial cells are sufficiently mobile to allow translocation of the cells so that with extreme distention the cell layer may become only a single one. There are normally no glandular or secreting cells within the vesical mucosa. The human bladder mucosa is a nonabsorptive and nonsecreting surface for all practical purposes.

This epithelium rests upon a loosely arranged tunica propria. The free use in the literature of the terms "submucosa" and "corium" is admissable if the meaning remains clear. The "corium" refers to the more dense superficial investment of the mucosa and the "submucosa" to the looser deep layers of tunica propria.

The tunica propria is indeed an astounding layer. It provides mobility for the mucosa by adapting to stretch. It apparently serves for the firm attachment of muscular fibers (e.g., some of the intrinsic longitudinal musculature of the ureter, the vesicocervical fibers in the region of the verumontanum and the prostatourethral fibers in the membranous urethra). It also contains smooth-muscle fibers with no other source of origin as far as detrusor connections are concerned, attached to the mucosa of the trigone and supramontane urethra. Its connective-tissue components are composed of loosely arranged collagen with very few elastic fibers and a diffuse and rich supply of blood vessels.

The tunica propria of the sphincteric urethra is quite different from that of the bladder. In the region of the trigone it loses its loosely arranged character and the corium of the mucosa rests upon the dense, fine-fibered myoelastic tissue of the longitudinal musculature of the vesicocervical system (superficial trigonal muscle). There are numerous thin-walled vascular spaces in this region which have been likened to erectile tissue, although they probably are more important in cushioning the sphincteric system and in local nutrition than in "erection." There are also small glandular structures in the female vesical neck which are the analogues of the cranial prostate in the male.[100a] Nerve endings within the tunica propria and mucosa are more prominent in the region of the trigone and vesical neck.

The distribution of smooth muscle and its histological configuration vary in different areas of the bladder and in the sphincteric urethra. In the vertex of the bladder, there are fewer elastic and collagen fibers than in the densely elastic layers of the membranous and inframontane regions of the male urethra. The elastic and collagen net of the superficial trigonal muscle is represented by closely packed, fine laminar sheets about the smooth-muscle cells.

In the dome of the bladder, individual muscle bundles are separated from one another by septa composed almost entirely of crisp collagen, with only a few scattered elastic fibers. These major septa are not only supports for the bundles and sources of the collagen septa which isolate the individual fascicles within the bundle but also provide the coarse matrix for the rich vascular, lymphatic and neural network necessary to the individual smooth-muscle cell (Fig. 26). Fascicles within a single bundle number from 3 to more than 20, and each contains an estimated 8 to 50 smooth-muscle cells. Each fascicle contains one or more centrally located capillaries 10 to 15 μ in diameter. The cytolemma of each smooth-muscle cell within a fascicle forms a mosaic pattern, staining strongly with PAS.

Individual smooth-muscle cells vary somewhat in diameter on transverse section. Some are sectioned in the region of the nucleus and show a clear space surrounding the nuclear membrane. The cytoplasm shows a fibrillar, ground-glass appearance, but myofibrils are not identifiable in their entirety. In fixed specimens the smooth-muscle cell presents the appearance of a spindle. Nuclei in fixed sections are centrally located within the cell and have the shape of attenuated ellipses. The nuclear membrane is prominent, there are one or two nucleoli, the chromatin is delicate and the nuclei are generally pale. In contracted cells the nuclei may show wrinkling and increased density so that, casually observed, they resemble reticular fibers or fragmented elastin.

Lymphatics within the collagenous septae of the muscular coats are normally small and accompany the vascular bundles. One or two delicate channels are usually noted accompanying the larger vessels; they are invariably smaller than either the artery or vein.

The varying proportions of smooth-muscle, collagen and elastic

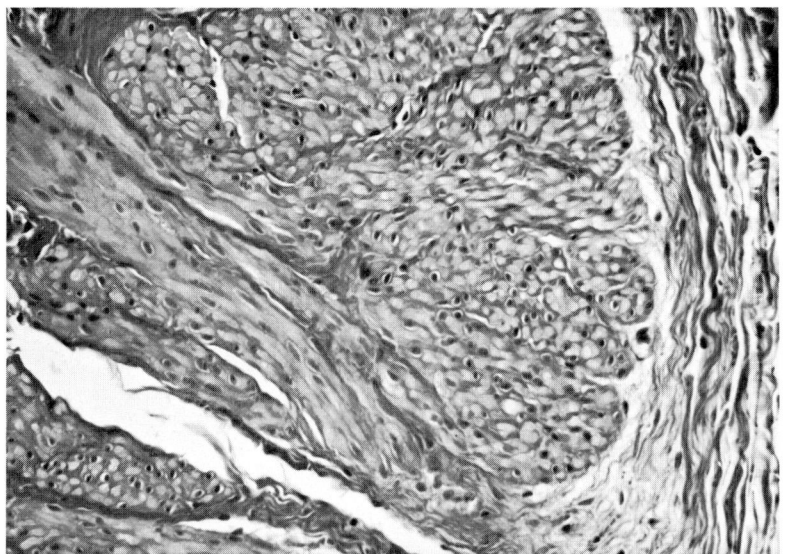

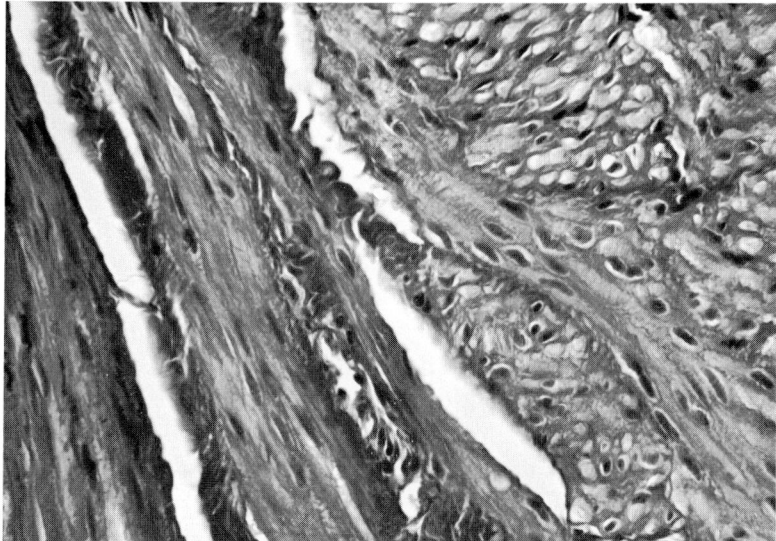

FIG. 26. Smooth muscle of the detrusor sectioned transversely, obliquely and longitudinally. Perimysial and endomysial compartmentation is seen in A. Smooth-muscle cell borders are intimately apposed. Note reticular fibers within the fascicle at left in B, and also the small capillary. Perimysial connective tissue is almost entirely collagen. Biopsy specimen from dome of bladder in a 3-year-old girl. Verhoeff-van Gieson stain. Original magnification X250 and X400.

fibers, each with its own degree of elasticity, alter the functional potential of the various regions of the bladder. Therefore, the walls of the bladder have reduced amounts of the most rigid elements, allowing the bladder to distend with its major component of smooth muscle. The walls of the sphincteric urethra, on the other hand, are more adapted to close occlusion with a preponderance of collagenous and elastic elements[560] as well as an added layer of striated muscle.

These tissue component balances may be altered with repeated extension cycles, prolonged distention, disease processes and age, so that the composite optimum elasticity of a particular region can become so altered that its function is impaired. Hypertrophy of smooth muscle accompanied by elastosis can take place in response to additional stress and compensate for minor degrees of detrusor imbalance. With aging there may be degeneration of collagenous and elastic tissue elements and the production of a considerable degree of urethral rigidity, particularly in the female,[433] which is incompatible with adequate sphincteric function.

It is interesting that the walls of the seminal vesicles are invested with a heavy layer of smooth muscle in a roughly circular distribution and a lighter outer coat of longitudinal smooth muscle. Elastic tissue here is dense in the submucosa and is even more so in the walls of the vas deferens and verumontanum. On the basis of light microscopy studies, it has been suggested that smooth muscle represents a syncytium.[286,368] Caesar, Edwards and Ruska in 1957[73] found no evidence of intercellular bridges in their electron microscopy studies of the urinary bladder and gallbladder of the mouse. Mark,[340] Thaemert[493] and Bergman,[21] however, hold that protoplasmic connections exist between smooth muscle cells. Thaemert[494] has presented electron microscopic evidence of what he terms "anastomotic intercellular bridges" between smooth-muscle cells, to emphasize their protoplasmic continuity (Fig. 27).

Thaemert has pointed out irregularly distributed, dense thickenings of the plasma membrane of the smooth-muscle cell in his electron photomicrographs, where there seemed to be a concentration and attachment of neighboring collagen fibrils. In no instance has there been noted penetration of the plasma membrane by either collagen or elastic fibrils.

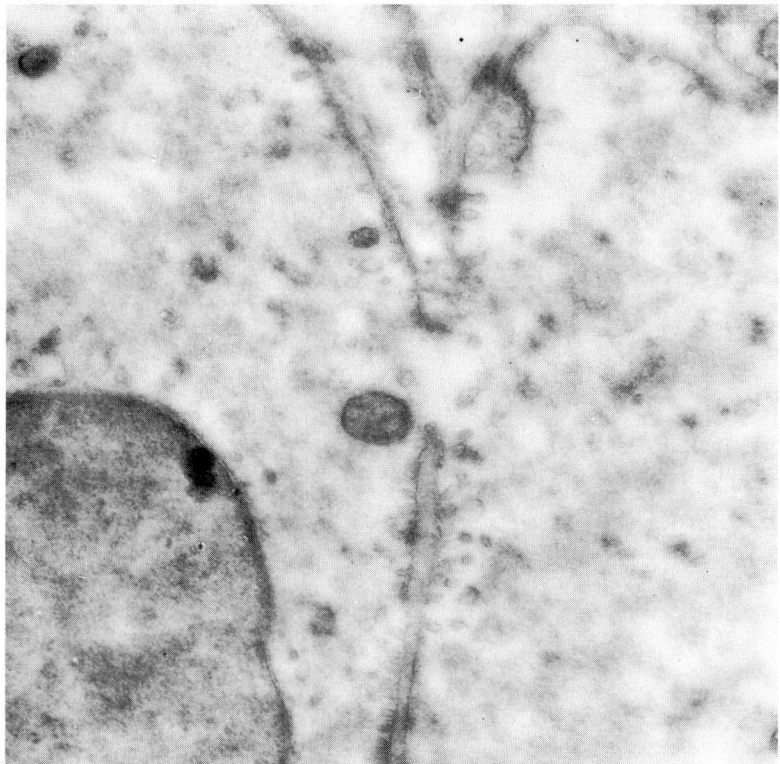

FIG. 27. Electron microscopic photomicrograph of smooth-muscle cell of rat intestine to show continuity of plasma membranes of two adjacent cells. This continuity provides for protoplasmic anastomosis of the two cells. X30,000. (Courtesy of J. C. Thaemert.)

In sections of the bladder and sphincteric urethra stained with Masson's trichrome (Goldner modification), Verhoeff-van Gieson and Luxol fast-blue-PAS and examined with the light microscope, there is a clear tinctorial differentiation among the smooth-muscle, striated-muscle, collagen and elastic fibers. Examination of the intrinsic striated sphincter, although revealing a rich mixture of smooth and striated muscular elements, fails to reveal any direct syncytial relationship between the two types. The collagen and elastic fibers intertwine among the muscle fascicles, and it is presumably by mutual attachments to these that the important connections between smooth and striated muscles are effected in the sphincteric system. These connections would seem to qualify eminently for the name of "petits tendons" which has been applied to them.

The insertions of the posterior bandelette fibers into the trigone provide another variation of this type of force transmission in which histologically transversely sectioned smooth-muscle fibers bear a similar relationship to the longitudinal ones. The nature of these tendinous attachments on an ultrastructural level presents an intriguing concept and deserves much further study.

ELASTIC AND COLLAGEN COMPONENTS

Normally occurring elastic fibers associated with collagen are found throughout the bladder musculature and are arranged as a supporting web for the smooth-muscle fibers. With light microscopy, the nature of the contacts between the smooth-muscle cells and these fiber elements is indistinct. Electron microscopy offers evidence that there is some type of fibrocellular adherence,[456,116] rather than simply a joint embedding of the diverse elements in a common ground substance.

The tunica propria of the more distensible portions of the bladder contains a few elastic fibers and quite loosely organized collagen fibers. There are no elastic tissue layers, nor is there evidence of specific organization of these fibers within the detrusor muscle. The collagen-elastic meshwork in general parallels the smooth-muscle bundles and fascicles and appears to be laid down along the lines of force proscribed by the smooth-muscle bundles.

In the superficial trigonal muscle, the first intimation of a difference in the fiber pattern becomes evident. Except for the "corium" of the mucosa, the tunica propria is, for all practical purposes, absent. The mucosa lies directly upon a regimented, longitudinal array of elastic and smooth-muscle fibers, both of which appear to be elongated, closely packed and precisely oriented from the interureteric ridge toward their gathering at the vesical neck and subsequent insertion at the verumontanum. Both the smooth-muscle fibers and the elastic fibers appear to be smaller in diameter in both longitudinal and cross sections. This appearance is probably due merely to their elongation and compression in this tissue layer. There is an increase in the amount of elastic tissue in this layer, and the elastic fibers seem to be more closely applied to the smooth-muscle cells than they are in the detrusor musculature.

The collagen of the "corium" of the mucosa in which the epithelial cells are imbedded can be seen as fine branching processes within the mucosal folds. This pattern of mucosa resting directly upon "myo-elastic tissue" is present throughout the sphincteric urethra, but is not as prominent in the anterior and lateral vesicocervical smooth-muscle bundle system at the vesical neck as it is in the superficial trigonal muscle.

In the midurethra, cross sections including the verumontanum show a definite and constant distribution of elastic fibers. A definite and firmly packed layer of collagen and elastic fibers is seen bracketing the floor of the urethra approximately 20 to 30 μ beneath the mucosa. These fibers surround the urethra, but thin out laterally and anteriorly. The verumontanum shows extensions of this fibroelastic layer sweeping upward within its summit.

McCarthy, Ritter and Klemperer[364] have suggested that the presence of elastic tissue in the verumontanum is related to the ejaculatory ducts (Fig. 28). The inframontane urethra is especially dense with elastic fibers. The same elastic layer which sweeps into the verumontanum is seen in longitudinal section to course into the membranous and bulbous urethra dorsally in company with the prostatourethral smooth-muscle bundles, giving up numerous branching slips to form the submucosal elastic arc in the membranous urethra described by Pennington and Lund.[396]

In cross section there is an interesting relation between this deep elastic bracket and the circular smooth muscle of the inframontane urethra. The longitudinal prostatourethral bundles are immediately surrounded by elastic slips. Then the ventral circular smooth muscle fascicles, as they thin out posterolaterally, are met and actually interlace with branching cords of elastic fibers, the nether ends of which are continuous with the heavily elastic core of the verumontanum, crista urethralis and ejaculatory duct systems. It is not inconceivable that the force of smooth-muscle contraction during ejaculation could be transmitted through these interdigitations.

The female urethra shows no such layer of elastic fibers, either in the tunica propria or beneath the innermost smooth-muscle layers.

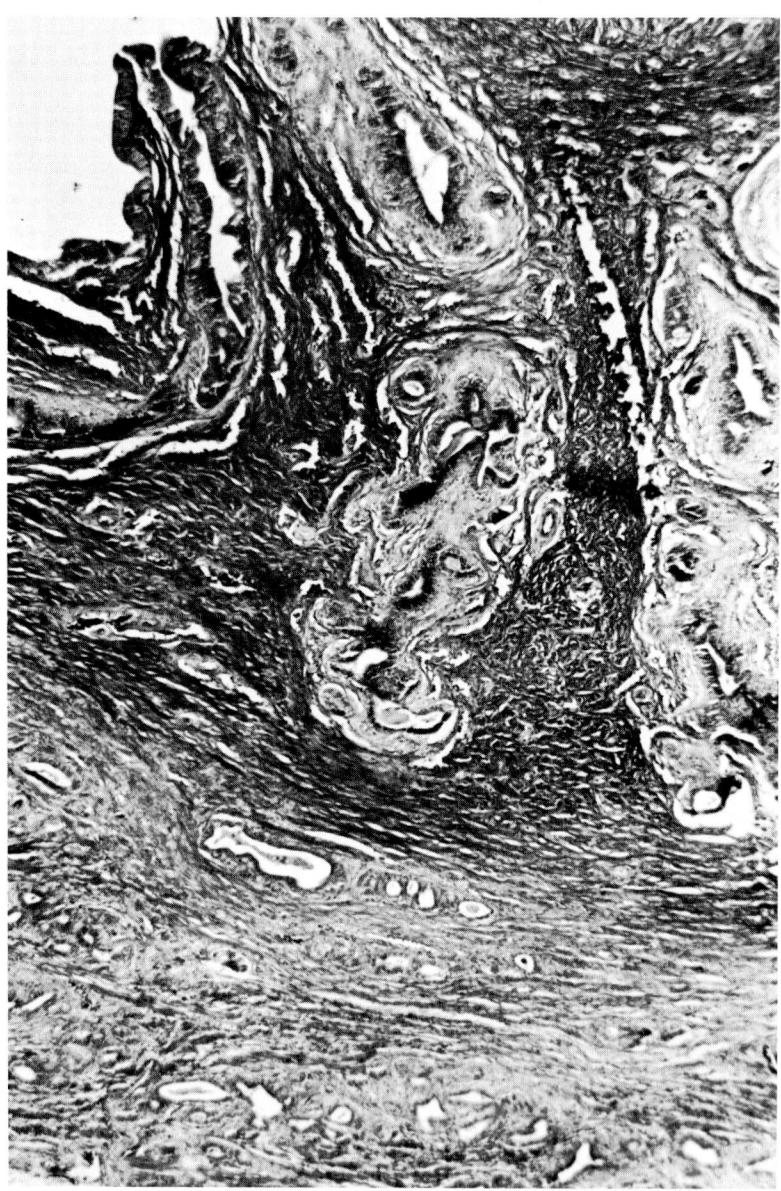

FIG. 28. Distribution of elastic fibers in the tunica propria and verumontanum in a 6-year-old male.

There is, indeed, very little elastin to be seen, even between the smooth-muscle bundles. The fibers noted are discrete, associated with collagen, and show the random distribution seen throughout the detrusor musculature. Pennington and Lund found a significant concentration of elastic fibers only between the intrinsic striated-muscle bundles of the sphincter in the female urethra.

III

Physiology of Micturition

Muscular Mechanisms of Urination

An unresolved problem in our thinking of the mechanism of urination and continence has been the concept that a sphincter must relax reciprocally in response to the expulsive force of a hollow viscus. The classical animal experiments of Learmonth (1931),[309] Elliott (1907),[134] Langworthy, et al. (1939-1940)[292, 293] and Denny-Brown and Robertson (1933)[113] tended to support this concept.

There is now anatomical and neurophysiological evidence in both animals and humans to permit some revision of this view.[299, 553, 145, 173, 174, 489, 273, 37]

Reciprocal inhibition cannot be totally disregarded, however. Electromyographic evidence shows electrical silence in the striated perineal musculature of the human "external sphincter" during urination.[157, 399, 246] There is also a resurgence of interest in the functional significance of the sympathetic innervation of the trigone. The specific mechanisms here are still elusive.

Anatomically, the process of urination can be considered to be a predominantly parasympathetically controlled, positive contraction of the smooth-muscle elements of the bladder and sphincteric urethra, in which the sphincteric urethra is actively drawn open in a radial fashion by longitudinal smooth-muscle elements with origins in the detrusor.[172, 173, 244, 299, 487] Woodburne,[553] working on a gross anatomical level, believed that the muscle bundles of the detrusor arched away from the vesical neck to accomplish this.

S. Gil Vernet[171] has shown, however, that there is actual *insertion* of the longitudinal smooth-muscle bundles into the trigone, the mucosa of the urethra and the intrinsic striated portion of the urinary sphincter. These fiber bundles, acting in concert with the expulsive force of the detrusor, serve to funnel the vesical neck and to draw aside the arcuate vesical-neck smooth muscle, and perhaps the intrinsic striated musculature as well. This accounts clearly for the shortening and widening of the urethra which have been observed experimentally in dogs[295] and clinically in humans.[301, 272, 318, 244, 245]

Histotopographic sections show striated muscle to extend to the vesical neck ventrally in both male and female and to have connections with smooth-muscle bundles within the posterolateral portions of the trigone.[221, 201, 330, 34, 224, 339] In addition, striated muscle forms a circular ring in the membranous male urethra, and in the middle third of the female urethra. At all of these sites there is an intimate connection of smooth and striated muscle cells, sometimes apparently mediated by connective tissue bridges. Such a tissue connection has been postulated by numerous authors.[521, 293, 440] This is in accord with Bors'[37] concept of the synergistic action of smooth and striated muscles in the urinary sphincter.

The intrinsic striated sphincter in the male may serve for the expulsion of semen during ejaculation with the circular and arcuate smooth-muscle bundles of the montane and inframontane urethra. Hutch[243, 244] has postulated an *opening* mechanism for the intrinsic striated sphincter in which the entire perineal musculature presumably takes part. Bors[33] has demonstrated weak contractions of the vesical neck with pudendal nerve stimulation in human paraplegics. Paradoxically, Lapides, et al.[296, 297, 298] and Petersen, Kjellberg and Dhuner,[400] in their studies of pudendal nerve blockade with systemically administered curare and succinylcholine, demonstrated that urination can occur without the aid of *any* of the perineal striated musculature. Krahn and Morales[281] found no incontinence, nor even decrease in urethral resistance, in postprostatectomy patients following pudendal nerve blocks, despite the fact that in some patients the internal portion of the sphincteric system had been destroyed. These observations would seem to indicate that the striated muscles of the pelvic floor (levator ani, bulbocavernosus, ischiocavernosus and transverse perineal) have little to do with the initiation of urination or resting continence under normal circumstances.

It has been generally assumed that the function and structure of the *intrinsic* striated sphincter are the same as those of the striated muscle of the perineum generally. Physiological measurements of the anal sphincter and levator ani muscles are presumed accurately to reflect the function of the intrinsic striated sphincter.[246,490,158,399] It should also be considered that the intrinsic striated musculature of the sphincteric urethra may have a different type of innervation, and possibly a different physiological response.[175,549]

Anatomically, the only relationship between the intrinsic striated sphincter and the perineal musculature is the rather minor connection in the region of the rectourethralis confluence. The intrinsic striated sphincter may function somewhat independently of the perineal striated musculature and in a closer synergism with smooth muscle. It seems probable that it assists in closure of the proximal urethra at the end of micturition, by virtue of its lateral subtrigonal smooth-muscle connections and circular disposition in the membranous urethra.

Functionally, the smooth musculature of the vesical neck and sphincteric urethra can be considered as two antagonistic groups, the *retentive* and the *expulsive* (Fig. 29). Those muscle bundles and tissues with a largely *retentive* function are: (1) the detrusor loops and the trigonal loop acting as obliquely opposed arcs at the vesical neck; (2) arcuate ventral smooth muscle of the membranous urethra; (3) the intrinsic striated sphincter; (4) the dense dorsal elastic submucosal arc (Pennington's arc) in the membranous urethra; and (5) the submucosal mesh of collagen, elastic fibers and vascular spaces throughout the sphincteric urethra which transmit the periurethral muscular forces to the lumen and effect a cushioned coaptation of the mucosa.[554]

At resting lengths, these structures perform a minimum of metabolic work and their effectiveness as water-tight sphincters is the net result of their meshed tonus and elasticity, arranged as they are in a mutually complementary anatomical distribution.

The *expulsive* group, that is, those muscular elements responsible for the initiation and maintenance of urination, includes: (1) the de-

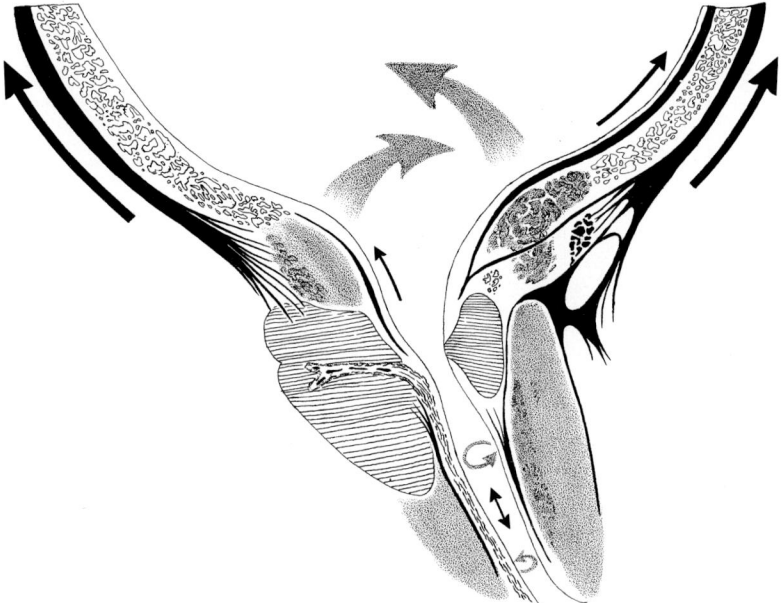

FIG. 29. Diagram to show the presumed function of the various muscle bundles of the sphincteric urethra. The direction of contraction and relative forces are indicated by the size and orientation of the arrows. The muscle groups representing the forces of expulsion are indicated in black. Those representing arrest of urination are stippled.

trusor; (2) the longitudinal continuations of the detrusor into the sphincteric urethra, namely, the posterior lateral longitudinal bundle, the anterior and lateral longitudinal bundles of the detrusor, the vesicocervical, vesicoprostatourethral and prostatourethral systems and their analogues in the female, the vesicourethral and cervicourethral systems; (3) the posterior longitudinal bundle (bandelette); (4) the transverse precervical arc; and (5) the inner anterior longitudinal bundle.

During normal filling of the bladder, the intravesical pressure rises only very slightly until a voiding capacity is reached. The resting tonus of the arcuate retentive sphincteric system is sufficient to assure continence at these relatively low pressure levels. Probably only a small retentive role is played by the collapsed distal sphincteric urethra during the normal filling of the bladder. Clinically, a partially filled bladder demonstrated by cystourethrogram shows the contents to be arrested at the vesical neck (Fig. 30). In expulsion, the onset of

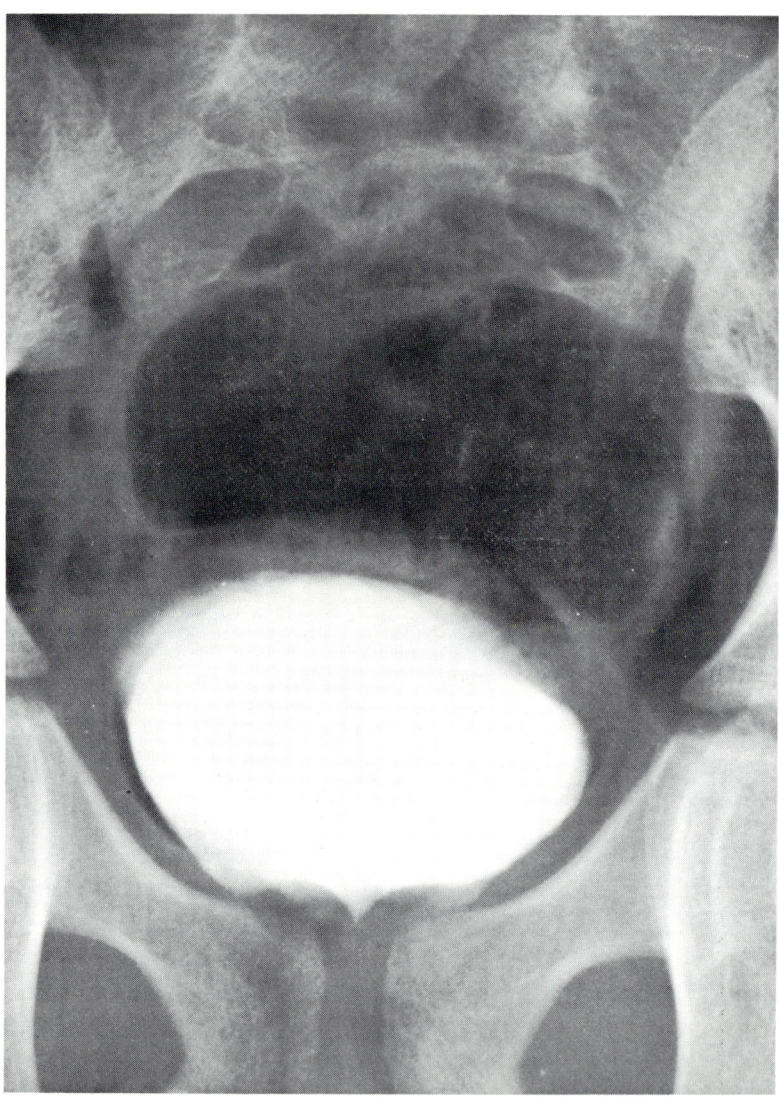

FIG. 30. Cystogram showing partially filled bladder at rest. Note the arrest of urine at the vesical neck. V-shaped beak at bladder base is due to occlusion at this point by the trigonal and detrusor loops.

micturition is dependent first upon *detrusor contraction*. At the moment of contraction, the longitudinal extensions of the detrusor throughout the sphincteric urethra actively draw aside the arcuate muscle bundles of the vesical neck to form the funnelled vesical neck, which is the hydrodynamically most favorable[335,336] (Fig. 31). The urethra is in this manner simultaneously widened and shortened. The powerful posterior longitudinal bundle elevates the trigone and posterior base of the bladder, further increasing the fetch of the funnel.[171,176,245,451]

The muscle fiber bundles acting simultaneously at this moment about the circumference of the vesical neck are the longitudinally disposed *vesicocervical fibers* (anteriorly and laterally) and the *posterior vesicocervical fibers* (superficial trigonal muscle). The latter, by means of their mucosal insertions in the region of the verumontanum, elongate the distal tip of the vesical-neck funnel by some assistant internal stretching of the vesical neck loops.

At the same time, the vesicoprostatourethral system contracts to open the inframontane and membranous urethra. The prostatourethral fibers exert their force, again circumferentially, on their mucosal attachments to the membranous urethra, slightly shortening the inframontane urethra. The vesicourethral fibers attached to the intrinsic striated sphincter may also assist in drawing the membranous urethra open centrifugally. It is suggested that the intrinsic striated sphincter undergoes some inhibition during micturition.* As long as the detrusor continues to contract, its extensions into the sphincteric urethra contract with it to maintain the open, funnelled urethra (Figs. 32*A*, *B*).

At the end of urination, the intrinsic striated sphincter contracts; the vesical neck closes (detrusor loop and trigonal loop) as the contraction of the detrusor diminishes and dies away over a few seconds. The longitudinal musculature of the sphincteric urethra lengthens in relaxation. The circular smooth muscle of the membranous urethra is allowed to contract similarly, as normal resting tonus is restored. The tissue tension of the elastic, vascular and collagen net can then be released to further obliterate the lumen of the urethra. At the vesical

---

*The electromyographic silence recorded by both intra-urethral needle electrodes and perineal electrodes is most intriguing. With arrest of urinary flow there is a resumption of the striated-muscle resting action potentials. Whether these studies actually reflect the intrinsic striated sphincter muscle itself or the surrounding perineal musculature is still not clear, and cannot be so until the innervation of the intrinsic striated sphincter is established.

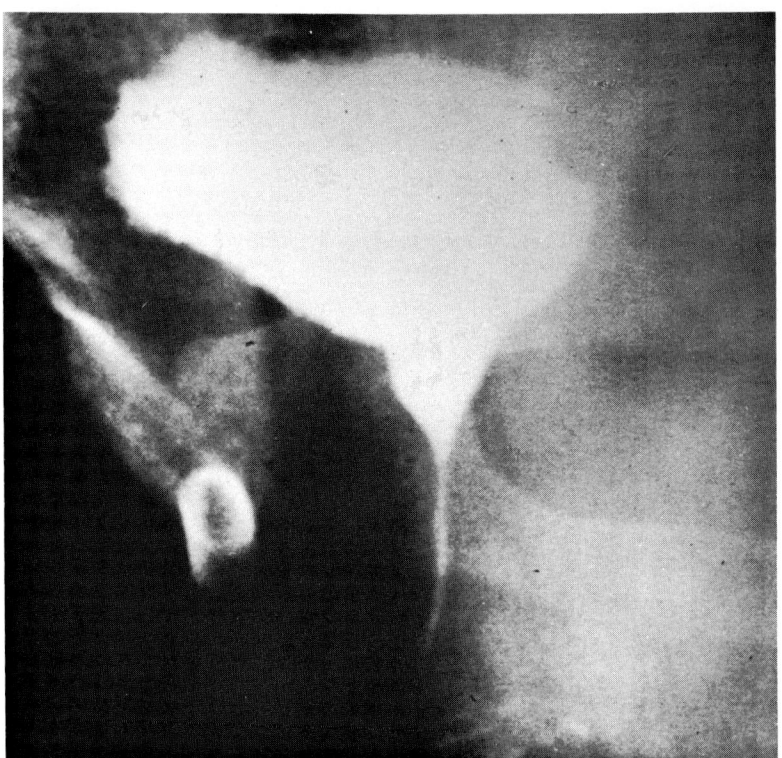
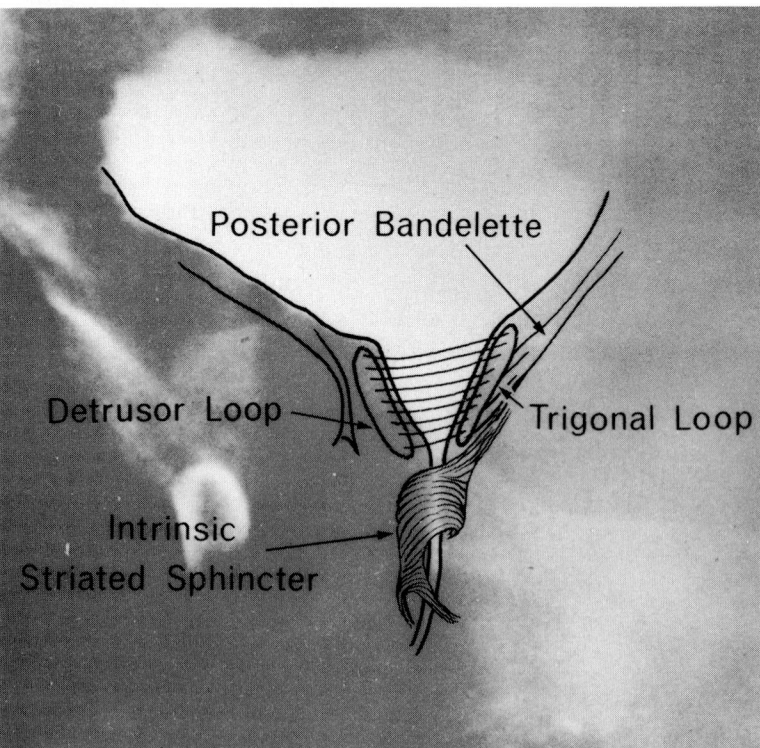

FIG. 31. Oblique voiding cystourethrogram to show funnelling of the vesical neck with the initiation of voiding. Overlay diagram (below) to show distribution of muscle bundles and their influence upon the luminal configuration.

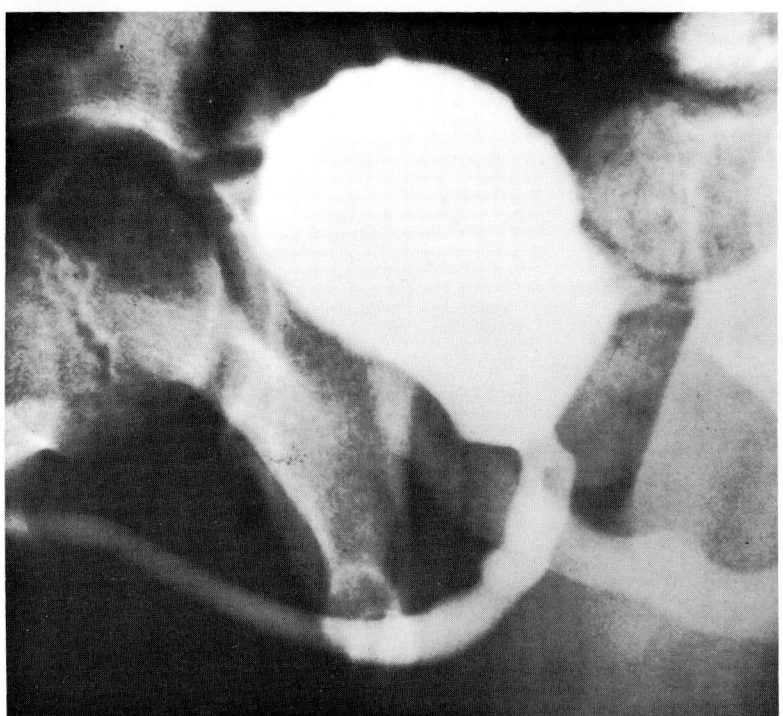
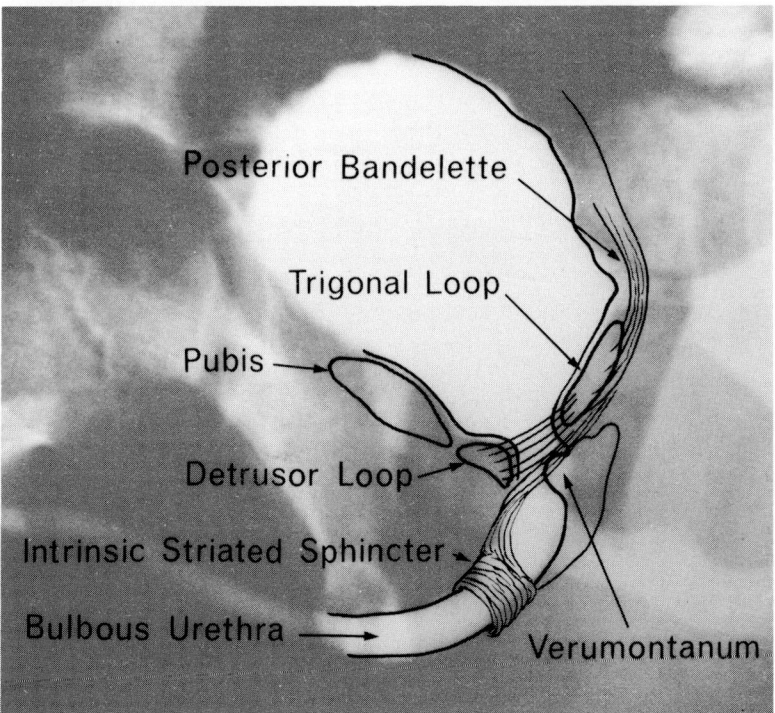

FIG. 32. *A*, Oblique voiding cystourethrogram in 6-year-old boy. Detrusor contraction produces irregular configuration of the fundus of the bladder. The base of the bladder is widely funnelled and smooth in luminal outline. This represents the "broken base plate" described by Hutch. Note the slight decrease in density of the contrast medium and indentations of the lumen at the sites of most dense circular and arcuate musculature (vesical neck and membranous urethra).

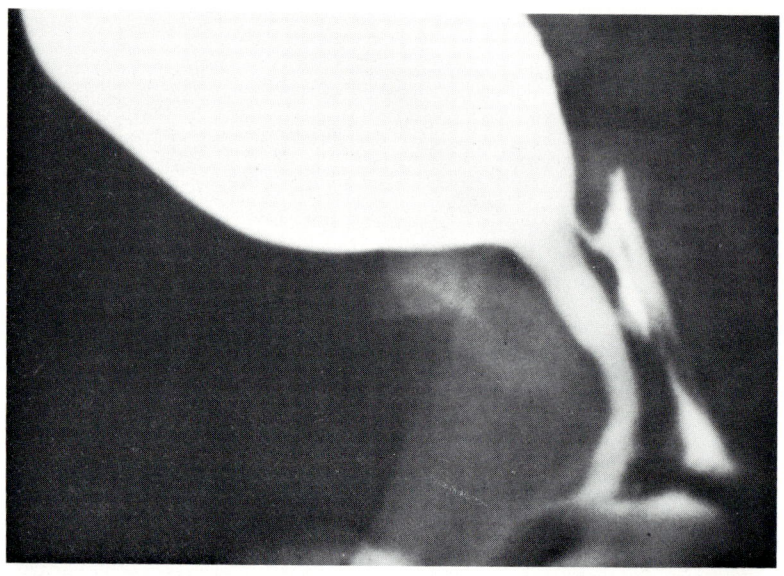

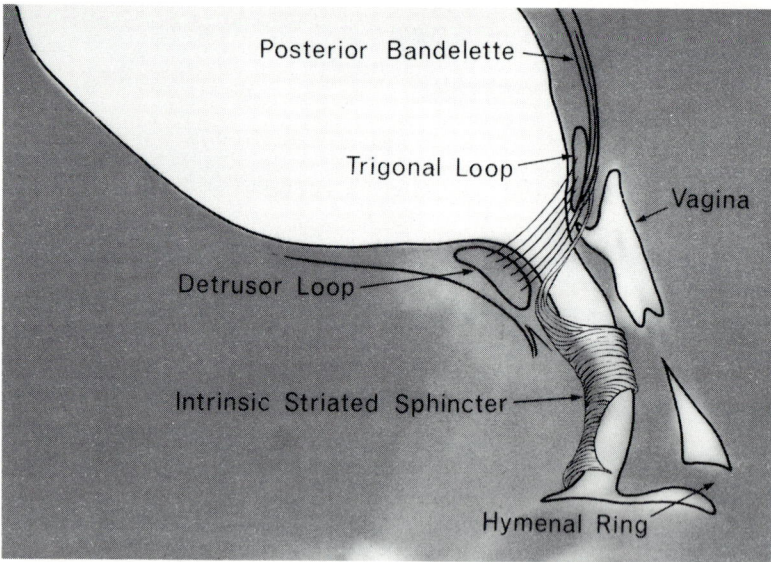

FIG. 32. *B*, Oblique voiding cystourethrogram in 8-year-old girl. Base plate is steeply canted. Vesical neck is funnelled. Note normal indentation and decrease in contrast density in middle third of the sphincteric urethra. This is the site of maximum investment by intrinsic striated sphincter. Vaginal reflux, a common finding, is evident.

neck, the cessation of active contraction of the posterior longitudinal bundle allows the bladder base in the adult to resume its resting, roughly right-angled relationship to the internal urethral orifice. The funnelled shortening and widening of the urethra, essential during micturition, have been reversed so that the funnelled neck disappears, the lumen is occluded and the resting length of the urethra restored.

It is important to realize that the shortening of the urethra during urination takes place largely in its proximal portion. The inframontane urethra and membranous urethra are relatively fixed, as is the distal urethral segment in the female. The previously noted "relaxation of the pelvic floor," which was believed necessary to precede urination, in all probability can be interpreted as the opening of the vesical neck on a somewhat grander scale than formerly imagined.

In summary, the smooth and striated vesicourethral musculature of the sphincteric urethra operates as an anatomical and functional unit. The voluntary striated muscle of the perineum comes into play only at the end of urination, at which time urine remaining within the bulbous urethra can be voluntarily stripped into the dependent pendu-ous urethra by the action of the bulbocavernosus and ischiocavernosus muscles.

Neuromuscular Mechanisms

Two columns of nerves from the hypogastric plexus course along the posterolateral borders of the vesical neck and prostate and emanate from the numerous perivesical dorsolateral ganglia in the region of the vesical neck, innervating the sphincteric urethral smooth muscle. They may also be importantly related to the ejaculatory function.

The three anterior columns have few gangliar interruptions in the perivesical plexus and may predominately supply the innervation to the sphincteric system. There are, of course, numerous connections among all of these longitudinal nerve columns, so that the prostate and membranous urethra are enmeshed in an autonomic (largely parasympathetic) collar. It is impossible to determine which fibers carry sensory or motor impulses, or both. Adrenergic and cholinergic ganglion cells and nerve endings have been demonstrated in the region of the trigone and vesical neck, but there is currently no study differentiating adrenergic and cholinergic nerve endings within the sphincteric urethra (Fig. 33).

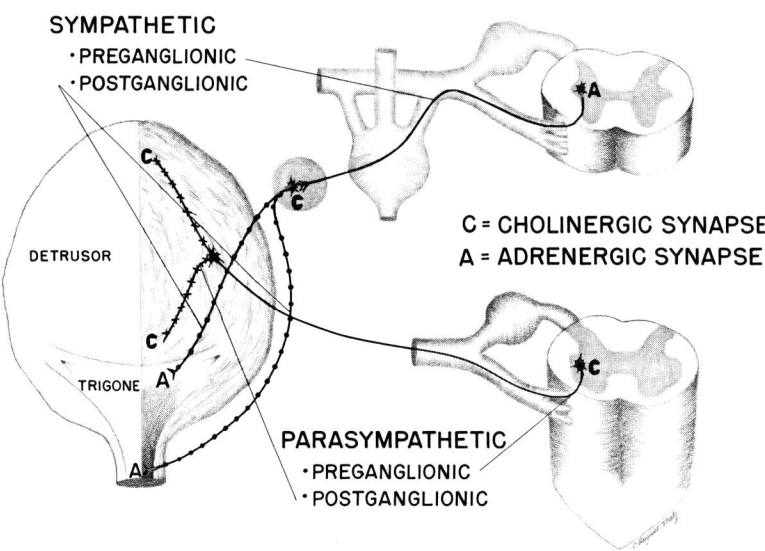

FIG. 33. Pathways of autonomic nerves and ganglia in the detrusor and trigone. (After Blanca Smith and Netter.)

The autonomic mucosal nerve endings in the trigone and vesical neck register pain, but not touch or thermal sensation.[35] Nesbit and Lapides,[374] Sabetian[448] and Bors and Blinn[36] have provided good evidence for the lack of participation of mucosal afferent-nerve endings in the maintenance of normal tonus of the bladder musculature. The stimulation of mucosal and submucosal afferent-nerve endings with irritant solutions produces a profound reflex micturitional response, but does not alter the intrinsic tonicity of the bladder musculature (Sabetian[449]). The tonus of the bladder wall is assumed to be primarily a myoelastic function under some degree of reflex control.[50,225]

This is not to say that detrusor tonus is a totally passive state. Smooth muscle has intrinsic rhythmicity,[404,278,491] as does cardiac muscle to a much greater extent, and an intercellular (either syncytial or cell-membrane transmitted) reflex transmission system may exist among smooth-muscle cells serving to adjust mural tension to intravesical pressures.

Central control in inhibition of urination has been the subject of much investigation and detailed description.[39,45,293,414,446,114] It is generally held that sensory fibers of the parasympathetic system are stimulated by stretch of the tunica propria and detrusor mesh, and

74 *Lower Urinary Tract Obstruction in Childhood*

impulses recording this event are transmitted to the sacral-cord segments of S_2, S_3 and S_4. Central notice is established via the spinal cord to the hypothalmus. Midbrain transmission and cortical recognition and response are subsequently established. The motor limb from the central reference again passes along the spinal cord and the efferent reflex arc of the parasympathetic nerves at the levels of S_2, S_3 and S_4, and is either completed or inhibited.

With progressive filling and distention of the bladder, the sensory limb of the reflex arc is increasingly bombarded with impulses. The cortical demand to urinate becomes insistent, and the motor limb of the parasympathetic outflow to the bladder is ultimately freed from its central inhibition and the detrusor and sphincteric urethra stimulated along the branches of the hypogastric plexus. The musculature of the entire bladder is stimulated in this view. There is as yet no demonstrable reflex inhibition of the sympathetic system in the human.

The response to this stimulation by the most powerful muscles of the detrusor can be visualized as overcoming the passive resistance of the opposed musculature. This is due primarily to a simple anatomical and mechanical advantage, as well as a considerably greater muscle mass. The question of exactly what happens to the parasympathetic impulses reaching the antagonistic musculature is still unanswered. It is difficult to believe that the intrinsic striated sphincter, the detrusor loops, trigonal loop and circular smooth muscle of the inframontane and membranous urethra act as if they were completely denervated. It is equally difficult to believe that they are inhibited by the same fibers which stimulate their counterparts. It seems reasonable to assume for the present that they are stimulated, but are unsuccessful competitors in the act of micturition.

Hutch[247] proposes, more specifically, that the rounded apogees of the detrusor loops (Heiss-Vernet) which are ventrally adherent to the overlying transverse precervical arc are actively pulled upward and forward by the insertion of the outer anterior longitudinal coat of the detrusor. The transverse precervical arc is tethered distally to the pubis by the pubovesical bundles, but despite this limitation there is some cranial displacement of the detrusor loops during voiding. The line of force of contraction of the detrusor loop is then diverted from its resting retentive arc at the vesical neck. Conceding stimulation of the detrusor loop with the rest of the bladder muscle, in this position its contraction becomes relatively ineffective due to its altered declination on the ventral slope of the widely funnelled vesical neck.

If, in fact, the intrinsic striated sphincter is also inhibited during micturition, the posterolateral subtrigonal striated connections may function to release the lateral limbs of the detrusor loop so that, together with the trigonal loop, they can respond to the upward pull of the posterior bandelette to form the dorsal half of the vesical neck funnel.

When the detrusor ceases to be stimulated by parasympathetic motor impulses, and the expulsive smooth-muscle fibers have reached their resting length, no further stretch impulses are transmitted to the sensory centers of the spinal cord and these fiber bundles come to rest. The "unsuccessful competitors," those bundles responsible for resting continence, previously having been stretched to permit the outflow of urine, are allowed, and perhaps even encouraged by their stretch-reflex responses, to contract in their own anatomically proscribed orbits to restore the resting, continent contour of the vesical neck.

Cellular Morphology of Smooth Muscle

The smooth-muscle cell, though related to striated and cardiac muscle cells and probably functioning in a somewhat similar manner, does show unique features both morphologically and functionally.[144]

The smooth-muscle cell has been investigated electron microscopically, primarily by Thaemert,[494,495,496] Shoenberg,[457] Caesar, Edwards and Ruska,[73] Mark,[340] Bergman,[21] Gansler,[165] Weinstein and Ralph,[530] and Panner and Honig.[389] Studies have been carried out in the human and rat uterus,[340] mouse urinary bladder,[73] rat ureter,[21] small bowel in rabbits,[432] pregnant rabbit uterus,[457] and in the gastrointestinal tract, arterioles and urinary bladder of rats.[494,495,350]

The smooth-muscle cell varies considerably in size and function among various species of animals and even in the same animal. The smooth-muscle cell of the human urinary bladder has not been fully studied morphologically.[88,251] Functional studies of mammalian smooth muscle indicate a wide variation in transmission and contractile systems among visceral, vascular and quasi-postural smooth muscles.[420,103] For this reason the smooth-muscle cell described here is a somewhat stylized version, but it serves as a point of departure and provides some correlative clues to the ultrastructure of the cell furnishing the contractile function to the urinary bladder.

Difficulties have been experienced by both light and electron microscopists in measuring smooth-muscle cells in their contracted and extended states. Cells from the rat ureter were reported by Bergman to measure 500 μ long by 7 μ in diameter. Shoenberg found the cells of the rabbit uterus to be 55 to 70 μ long and 3.5 to 4 μ wide, but at the end of pregnancy to have enlarged to 103 to 135 μ in length and 4 to 8 μ in diameter.

The nucleus of the smooth-muscle cell is described as an elongated structure containing granules and one or two nucleoli. It has been measured from 0.013 mm to 0.080 mm in length and usually appears in the center of the cell. The nucleus is enclosed by a double membrane with thicknesses of 9 to 11 μ, separated by a space approximately 13 μ in width. There may be nuclear pores. The chromatin assumes a peripheral distribution.

The sarcoplasm of the smooth-muscle cell contains mitochondria, endoplasmic reticulum, Golgi complexes, vesicles of various sizes and granules of ribonucleic acid (RNA) associated with the endoplasmic reticulum (Mark,[340] Shoenberg,[457] and Gansler[165]). One identifying feature of the smooth-muscle cell is the presence of numerous ovoid, thin-walled vesicles 60 μ in diameter beneath the plasma membrane; these are thought to be pinocytotic vesicles and responsible for some of the cell's nutrition in the absence of an extensive capillary supply (Caesar, et al.[73]).

The demonstrable contractile elements in the cell consist of oblique and longitudinally arranged filaments with a diameter of 50 to 80 Å or about the size of the actin filaments in striated muscle.[457,209] The myofilaments are not necessarily parallel to one another and cannot be followed for any great distance.[340,372] There is no regular hexagonal arrangement of the filaments, nor is there evidence of a constant interfibrillary distance or cross connection between filaments which is observed in striated muscle.[211,208,250] Patches of dense material, possibly myosin, with a diameter of 250 Å distributed irregularly among the filaments have been identified.[209]

Actin and myosin can be isolated from smooth muscle by chemical means.[23] The content of actomyosin increases in the rabbit uterus during pregnancy,[102,371,372] and decreases with atrophy of the muscle or castration. The smooth-muscle concentration of actomyosin is lower than that of striated muscle as is its content of adenosine triphosphate (ATP) and adenosine triphosphatase.

The cytolemma (sarcolemma) of the smooth-muscle cell is composed of a basement membrane 9 to 25 μ thick, an interspace of 9 to 13 μ and an outer plasma membrane 7 to 11 μ thick.[73] Smooth-muscle cell membranes interdigitate with one another and their surfaces exhibit profiles of protrusions which occur as knobs, spikes and ridges. These protrusions are believed to serve as means of intercellular adherence.[350, 493, 116]

There has been much interest in the attachment of the contractile elements of the cell to the inner surface of the cell membrane. Mark in 1956,[340] though he was unable to demonstrate any definite connections, concluded that despite the longitudinal arrangement of the filaments and their presence in the terminal ends of the cell the force of contraction was not necessarily longitudinal, and that it could be exerted over a great area of the cell surface rather than concentrated at the pointed ends. Rosenbluth[441] in 1965 described electron-dense patches on the inner surface of the plasma membrane of smooth-muscle cells in toads. Obliquely aligned filaments within the cell appeared to have connections with these sites. The dense bodies in this species are probably paramyosin, but a contraction model could be postulated in which the interaction of myosin and actin exerted an angled tension along the longitudinal axis of the cell. More recently, Harman, O'Hagerty and Byrnes[213] described roughened spots on the inner plasma membrane which they labeled "grapple plaques" and which appeared to serve as sites of attachment for the longitudinal myofilaments within the smooth-muscle cell. They further noted derangements in the "grapple plaques" and myofilament attachments in achalasia of human esophageal smooth muscle.

Panner and Honig, in 1967,[389] proposed that all of the longitudinal myofilaments were actin, and that myosin existed in a relatively desegregated form as *dense bodies* or membrane-dense patches which were adherent to actin filaments. These are the presumed points of attachment of actin and myosin and analogous to the sarcomeres of striated muscle. The model of contraction which they propose is one in which the actin filaments interdigitate and slide with respect to one another, driven by small units of myosin.

Protoplasmic anastomoses found occurring between smooth-muscle cells of the gastrointestinal tract and arterioles of the rat are cylindrical in form and contain cytoplasm with a density similar to that of the connected cellular regions. The membranes of the connections were seen to be continuous with the membranes of the connected cells. Thickenings of the plasma membrane on some of the cytolemmal protrusions are interpreted as points of attachment to surrounding collagen or elastic fibers and adjacent cells. Other protrusions are found to lie in close contact to nerve endings. Where the plasma membranes of the axon and smooth-muscle cell are closely apposed, pre- and postsynaptic vesicles are present and there are numerous mitochondria within the cytoplasm of the smooth-muscle cell. This structure conforms to that of nerve endings in striated muscle and that within the central nervous system and autonomic ganglia. Thaemert concludes that these are the functional neuromuscular junctions.[495]

A further difference in the structure of smooth muscle, when compared with striated muscle, lies in the haphazard arrangement of its sarcoplasmic reticulum.

Reger[428] was able to identify cisternae, triads and transverse canals in earthworm smooth muscle. Peachy and Porter[395] related the sarcoplasmic reticulum in *striated muscle* to rapid transverse transmission of myofibril stimulation by virtue of the well developed system of transverse sarcotubules. This is in contradistinction to the poorly developed system of sarcotubules in smooth muscle which, it is reasoned, being a cell which contracts and relaxes slowly, does not need a rapid transmission system.

Porter[411] in 1961 and Porter and Palade[410] attribute the spread of excitation waves through the sarcoplasm of the *striated* muscle cell to the transverse system of sarcotubules so that almost simultaneous stimulation of the myofibrils is achieved. Measurements of the time required for contraction and relaxation in smooth muscle are compatible with an impulse system that spreads by diffusion throughout the cell to stimulate the individual myofibrils rather than dependence upon a sarcoplasmic reticular net. This *diffusion theory* of excitation was proposed by Bozler[41,43] and is supported by the observation that the waves of excitation have a velocity too slow for any known nerve conduction, and by evidence that both excitability and conduction were unchanged when ganglion-free preparations were used or abolished by the application of tetracaine or atropine to block all nerve conduction.

Prosser[418,419] makes an important functional distinction among types of smooth muscle. One is the *multi-unit* smooth muscle (pilomotor, nictating membrane and some blood vessels), which is incapable of independent activity and is activated entirely by nerves, is relatively insensitive to quick stretch and is not spontaneously rhythmic. At the other extreme is *unitary* smooth muscle (occurring in some portions of the viscera, the uterus and the ureter), which is largely spontaneously active, shows interfiber conduction, and is stimulated by quick stretch to contract. The unitary smooth muscle, though capable of independent activity, may be regulated as well by intrinsic and extrinsic nerves. The bladder and vas deferens display a combination of these two types of smooth muscle.

Prosser notes that, although conduction in unitary smooth muscle occurs from fiber to fiber, transmission is probably not based on mechanical *pull* from cell to cell. Support for this view comes from the fact that the speed of interfiber conduction occurs at a few centimeters per second in the long axis of the fiber and at a few millimeters per second in the transverse axis. From this standpoint it is interesting that Prosser should suggest the possibility of *differences* in the mechanical and electrical properties of the detrusor muscle and those of the internal and external sphincter mechanisms.

The electrophysiology of smooth muscle is considerably beyond the scope of this study and is, at best, incompletely understood in the human urinary bladder. Ureteral smooth muscle in experimental animals has received some serious attention.[416,417,253,275,276,69,70,71] Boyarsky,[39] Bradley and Teague[46,47] and Weinberg[529] have made major efforts to translate basic generalized knowledge of smooth muscle to the function of the ureter and detrusor muscle in the human. The obvious problem is again that of variation in type, responsivity and transmission, not only of the smooth muscle of the urinary tract but of the subtle variations in its contractile modalities within the calyces, renal pelvis, ureter, detrusor and sphincteric urethra.

A few generalizations regarding the stimulation of smooth muscle are important. Bozler[42] demonstrated the presence of action potentials in visceral smooth muscle and indicated that these originated from pacemaker areas, and that the spread of these action potentials was myogenic. The resting potential in smooth muscle, which is extremely variable, is assumed to be largely dependent upon the concentration gradient of potassium ions across the cell membrane. This is not entirely so, as sodium and chloride are also contributors to the resting potential, and ion transport is mediated, as in striated muscle, by adenine nucleotides and by calcium and magnesium. The vital link between ionic flux and the mechanical coupling of actin and myosin to produce contraction of the smooth-muscle cell is still missing.

Contraction of visceral smooth muscle is preceded by a depolarization of the cell membrane. The mechanism of action of acetylcholine is assumed to involve depolarization of the cell membrane and, thus, an increase in frequency of the action potential discharge.[71] Epinephrine, on the other hand, produces relaxation of intestinal and myometrial muscle by *hyperpolarization* of the cell membrane and cessation of action potential discharge.[56]

Investigation of the electrical activity of the detrusor muscle has been largely related to the quest for a method of artificial electrical stimulation of the neurogenic bladder.[480,454,341,200,40,499,260,261] Here, mass response of sheets of smooth-muscle cells must be considered, despite the fact that our knowledge of the individual cell is limited. Fredericks, et al.[160] were able to correlate rapid spiking action potential discharges in the dog's bladder, stimulated by gradual filling, with contraction of the detrusor. Initial pressure increases at near-voiding threshold were associated with spiking in the *anterior* and *posterior* detrusor muscle. They noted that maximal spiking corresponded to the greatest voiding pressure and to the beginning of a sustained, integrated voiding response of the detrusor. Electropotential changes were quite marked at the anterior (ventral) vesicourethral angle during the onset of this maximum response.

In experiments designed to localize trigger points for detrusor stimulation in human paraplegics,[202] it has thus far been impossible to demonstrate the areas of receptivity and impulse distribution described for the dog bladder.[454,200]

Conway and Bradley,[99] to assess the spread of excitation of the detrusor muscle in the dog, ingeniously measured the electrical impedence between multiple electrodes inserted into the detrusor muscle at various sites and recorded the order and magnitude of contractility of the various regions of the muscle based upon the distance between the implanted electrodes (e.g., the greater the distance, the greater the impedence). They found that the first event upon reflex induction of contraction was a low-amplitude contraction of the *dorsal urethrovesical junction* followed closely by a contraction of the fundus occurring in the midline. The predominant change at the urethrovesical junction was *stretch* or *relaxation*. The peak amplitude of detrusor contraction occurred concurrently with the peak amplitude of relaxation of the urethrovesical junction.

How is excitation of smooth muscle in the human bladder brought about? Prosser[419] suggests four possibilities: (1) mechanical stretch from cell to cell, (2) excitation of action potentials among axons interdigitated between muscle fibers, (3) excitation by a neurohumoral transmitter agent, inducing permeability change in smooth-muscle cells, or (4) electrotonic interaction between electrically active and inactive cells.

Bradley and Teague[46] are inclined to agree with Prosser's third and fourth possibilities based upon their studies in the cat, indicating the importance of ultrastructural tight junctions (nexus) between smooth muscle cells demonstrated by Dewey and Barr,[116] although these have not been observed in human bladder muscle. In the overdistended rabbit bladder, dislocation of these plasma-membrane thickenings has recently been correlated with detrusor hypotonia.[321] Whether the "nexus" is a purely mechanical, or a functional, transmitter between smooth-muscle cells is unresolved. Bradley and Teague suggest that the best present evidence indicates spread of excitation by way of *transmitter release* at one or more neuromuscular junctions on individual muscle cells. Thaemert's demonstration of protoplasmic bridges between smooth-muscle cells perhaps indicates a possible route for a neurohumoral transmission system.

Enzymatic studies of the smooth muscle of the urinary tract have been quite limited. Wein, et al.[528] characterized the activity of a number of enzymes involved in energy production or otherwise utilized in the activity of normal bladder muscle in dogs. These authors were particularly interested in the investigation of the reported accumulation of glycogen in neurogenic bladder muscle.[438] Succinic dehydrogenase (SDH), adenosine triphosphatase, and phosphorylase were abundantly present in normal muscle. There was very little glycogen synthetase. Following denervation only phosphorylase activity was found to be diminished. Swaiman and Bradley[482] found a pronounced increase in creatine phosphokinase (CPK) activity in the bladders of newborn rabbits between the 5th and 7th day of postnatal life. This increase corresponded to a similar increase in detrusor contractile response and indicates a functional maturation of an enzyme system which transfers a high-energy phosphate bond from creatine phosphate to adenosine triphosphate, similar to that found to occur to skeletal muscle during contraction.

COLLAGEN

Smooth-muscle bundles within the detrusor are separated by septae composed largely of collagen. The normal perimysial and endomysial septae show fine, rather loosely arranged fibrils which would appear to have very little limiting effect upon the contraction of smooth-muscle bundles. Elastic fibers within these septae are quite sparse. In the normal bladder fundus, fibroelastic tissue is probably of minor significance. In pathological changes associated with developmental abnormalities, disease, aging, injury or postoperative wound healing, collagen and elastin may, together, represent the governing moiety of the entire detrusor contractile mechanism. Smooth muscle regenerates very poorly.[442]

Collagen fibrils seen by electron microscopy exhibit an extremely regular banded appearance with a recurrent pattern periodicity of about 640 Å. This pattern is apparently related to the side-chain structures attached to the polypeptide backbone. The banding in this instance does not present much of a clue to the central amino-acid sequence of the collagen molecule, but does speak for the molecular basis for the observed morphology. Ramachandran and Kartha, in 1954,[423] put forth a triple-helical basic molecular structure for the collagen protofibril consisting of three intertwined polypeptide chains, each of which has again a helical configuration.

The tropocollagen particle, which can be considered the molecule of collagen, has a length of about 3000 Å and a diameter of 14 Å, and presumably consists of a single three-chain protofibril of this length.

From a biochemical standpoint, only a few major features will be mentioned. The excellent survey of G. N. Ramachandran[442] is recommended.

The amino-acid composition of collagen is very similar for a wide range of mammalian species. It has been determined that glycine forms very nearly one-third of the amino-acid residues of the molecule, and proline and hydroxyproline together form about two-ninths of the total number of amino acids in mammalian collagen. The sulfur-containing amino acids are very few in collagen. Tyrosine and histidine form less than one percent of the residue.

ELASTIN

The elastic "fiber" as a component of connective tissue varies in its morphology throughout the body, and there is considerable evidence, both electron microscopic and chemical, to suggest that elastic tissue is not an homogeneous tissue element.[203] Fibers are quite easily seen in most locations, however, and have been extensively studied.[522, 156] In the elastin fiber, the protein fibrillar core is felt to be surrounded by a carbohydrate-rich sheath or cement substance termed "elastomucin."[205] Elastic tissue is widely distributed throughout the body at sites where elasticity is required: the media of arteries and veins, lungs, ligaments, and dermis. In all these sites elastic fibers are associated with collagen, and both fibrous elements are embedded in an amorphous ground substance. Elastin is birefringent, with a refractive index of 1,534. It is resistant to digestion by crystalline trypsin, boiling water, hot alkali, acid, or high concentrations of urea.

Staining characteristics of elastin are striking with the elastic tissue stains, acid-orcein and resorcinol-fuchsin (Weigert's stain). The fibers stand out clearly from the surrounding collagen as intense purple to blue-black in color. The ultrastructure of the elastic fiber according to Lansing, et al.[294] is represented by a fiber 4.25 μ in diameter, made up of four or more helically arranged fibrils 1 μ in diameter within a matrix that is optically the same as the fibril. There is, however, less than general agreement of this finding, some authors holding that there is no organized internal structure to elastic fibers.

There is some similarity in the amino-acid composition of collagen and elastin, in that a third of the amino-acid residues of each is proline and another third is glycine. Neither contains more than traces of cystine, tyrosine, histidine, or tryptophan. In this connection, it is well to point out that all which stains like elastin is not necessarily elastin. Degenerating collagen may take an orcein or resorcinol-fuchsin stain, but in enzymatic studies with elastase the dye-absorbing substance has been found to be *pseudoelastin*.

Collagen has a relatively high tensile strength, and its module of elasticity is found to be 1×10^9 dynes per cm^2. Elastin, on the other hand, has a low tensile strength, and its module of elasticity is 3×10^6

dynes per cm². Collagen, then, is more resistant to stretch than elastin, has a greater tendency to return to its prestressed length, and requires greater forces to rend it asunder.

The association of collagen and elastin in all sites acts as a two-phase material, with a combination of the characteristics of each element. In arteries subjected to excessive pressures, the initial component involved is the elastic fiber which responds to initially lower pressures. Only secondarily is the more rigid collagen involved. The synergistic nature of the two-tissue elements under stress is further postulated to involve a simultaneous distribution of the distending forces by the more supple elastic fiber to its neighboring collagen supports.

The elasticity of the elastin molecule may be due to its unique nature among fibrous proteins, in that it contains a high concentration of long-chain, nonpolar amino acids. Elastic fibers have properties akin to those of rubber, and in this respect the structure of elastin resembles that of the polyisoprene backbone of the rubber molecule.

Hydrodynamics

The characteristics of urinary flow and the measurement of pressures within the bladder and urethra have been widely investigated in an attempt to evaluate the sum of the functions of the component anatomical parts.[360, 161, 453, 183, 237, 229, 53] It seems important to know as much as possible about the nature of the expulsive forces and the resistances against which they must operate. A comparison of normal values with the values found in various states of disturbed function should then be possible.

Hydrodynamic study has been proposed as a potential diagnostic measure; however, detailed pressure-flow measurements have been found to be of more basic fundamental value than diagnostic significance. Pressure-flow measurements represent, on the whole, an estimate of tissue integrity, i.e., the innervation and contractility of the smooth muscle plus the supporting collagen-elastic mesh which together are responsible for the transport of the urine. *Voiding cystometry*, an excellent uncomplicated term suggested by Donahue and G. Leadbetter,[119] categorizes the nature of the clinical study quite well.

Voiding cystometry is by no means indicated in every case and cannot be expected to substitute for a careful history, observation, examination, radiography and endoscopy.[570,184,190,362,361] On many occasions the diagnosis and treatment are clearly evident with the urologist's conventional armamentarium.

From a clinical standpoint, the most important hydrodynamic measurement is the resistance presented by the sphincteric urethra to the outflow of urine from the bladder. The drop in pressure across the sphincteric urethra (the "pressure gradient") should be the simplest method of assessing this factor. This is relatively difficult to measure mechanically; for this reason, it is generally measured indirectly by the formula: resistance = pressure/flow.[178]

The pressure in this formula is that generated by the detrusor, and is called the intravesical pressure. The flow rate is in milliliters of urine expelled per second. When converted into units of force, resistance is expressed in dyne sec/cm^2 (Gleason and Lattimer, 1962).

Tension developed within the walls of the urethra and ureters has been measured with fluid and air-filled balloons connected to recording devices.[462,460,461,347] Schwartz and Brenner in 1922[452] measured intravesical pressure during voiding with an urethral catheter. Von Garrelts[24] credits Rehfisch (1897)[429] with the first significant attempt to measure intravesical voiding pressures (54 cm H$_2$O) and construct curves graphically representing pressure changes during micturition. Bonney in 1923[29] estimated sphincter resistance by forcing fluid into the bladder via the urethra and noting the pressure necessary to overcome the sphincteric mechanism. Major advances in the field awaited the simultaneous measurement of urethral pressures, flow rates and intravesical pressures by means of small catheters, transducers, telemetry, micromanometers and radioisotopes.[264,20,226,179,181,550,78,571,141,228] These systems can be immensely sensitive and largely atraumatic to the patient, so that a wide sampling of reliable normal and abnormal records has been obtained.

Computer analysis of the radiographic configuration of the sphincteric and distal urethra can be applied to measure the site of dissipation of bladder energy, and the "fluid energy loss" at these points correlated directly with resistance.[146]

Gleason and Bottaccini in 1968,[183] in their energy-loss studies in 15 female children, found that the maximum resistance (greatest energy loss) resided in the distal segment of the female urethra. The most obstructed urethra in their series showed an energy loss of a modest 12.4 percent of the total energy available to the urinary stream.

Their studies assumed a funnelled proximal urethra. The diameter of the distal segment (equal to the "vena contracta," which is the exit diameter of the fluid column where the velocity is nearly uniform and usually the greatest) measured between 2 mm and 3 mm in the children studied. Theoretically, minute changes in the diameter of the vena contracta can produce marked variations in the flow rate.

Whitaker and Johnston in 1966[533] developed a tambour device connected via a transducer with a recording mechanism which directly measured the exit velocity (in mm Hg) of the urinary stream at a variable but small distance from the urethral meatus.

Whitaker, Johnston and Lawson,[534] further refining their calculations and methods, established a standard of *normal urethral resistance* in girls as 0.0762 mm Hg per (ml per sec)^2. If resistance calculated from intravesical pressure and flow rate alone falls below this figure, the possibility of outflow obstruction can be excluded. A figure higher than this calls for the inclusion of the equivalent exit pressure (P_e) in their equations (calculated from the measured exit velocity (V_e)) to measure the remaining kinetic energy in the exiting stream. Thus, their expression of resistance is:

$$R = \frac{P_B - P_E}{F_2}$$

where R = resistance in mm Hg per (ml/sec)^2
P_B = pressure energy of bladder fluid at the beginning of micturition (in mm Hg)
F = rate of flow in (ml/sec)^2
P_E = the equivalent exit pressure in mm Hg.

Von Garrelts' original choice of significant vesical hydraulic measurements were: *resting pressure* (i.e., the intravesical pressure at volumes ranging from 73 cc to 456 cc in his studies), *maximum micturition pressure*, which is the highest pressure noted during an individual voiding, and *postmicturition pressure*, the intravesical pressure measured at the end of urination. In determining flow, he measured the *total volume* voided, the *micturition time* and calculated the *mean flow*.

Voiding cystometry has been combined with cineradiography.[570,550,503,14,479,533] Simultaneous electromyography of the "striated external sphincter" during micturition has been carried out by the intra-urethral insertion of needle electrodes and by their perineal placement.[141,246,157,399,14] These authors have recorded electrical silence in the perineal musculature during urination, and resumption of resting electrical potentials with voluntary interruption of the stream or upon the termination of urination. A similar occurrence has been demonstrated in the anal sphincter during urination.[79,246]

Indirect measurements of pressure and flow rates provide most of our knowledge of the function of the bladder and sphincteric urethra, but urethral resistance has also been determined directly. Enhorning[141] measured intra-urethral pressure in women at various levels in the urethra and found the greatest resistance to be between 19 to 96 cm of water at a point 1 to 1.5 cm distal to the vesical neck. Lapides, et al.[301] measured intra-urethral pressures with a small catheter at different levels and recorded the highest intra-urethral pressure in the middle 2.0-cm segment of the female urethra (presumed in its entirety to be 4.0 cm long). The pressure here was 46 to 51 cm of water. In the male a maximum pressure of 47 cm of water was recorded in the region of the membranous urethra.* It is somewhat simpler to calculate the resistance from the known intravesical pressure and maximum flow rate than to measure it directly.

Direct measurements are interesting from an anatomical standpoint and provide information about the nature of the muscular concentrations surrounding the urethra. The formula for calculation of urethral resistance presented by Zatz,[570] which takes into account the turbulent nature of urinary flow, friction, mural tension, luminal diameter and length, appears to be one of the simplest and best of these.

$R = P_t/Q$ where R is the urethral resistance, P is the maximal voiding intravesical pressure and Q the maximal flow rate in ml/sec.

Nunn and Stephens[383] reported a pressure gradient between the bladder and urethra in normal male children of 0 to 12 mm Hg. Female children with obstruction showed gradients of 20 mm Hg or more. The authors felt that children with gradients of 12 mm Hg or less were unlikely to have urethral obstruction.

King, Mellens and White[271] found the intravesical pressure rise during voiding (i.e., maximal voiding pressure minus resting pressure)

*100 cms H_2O = 73.529 mm Hg.

to be 40 mm Hg or less in normal subjects, with increases of greater than 60 mm Hg in patients with obstruction. Pressure gradients in most of their normal subjects were below 9 mm Hg and in most cases of obstruction were greater than 18 mm Hg. The elevation of pressure in their studies included increased intra-abdominal pressure.

A normal maximal flow rate of 15 ml/sec was established by Zatz for a group of female children regardless of age, and this figure appeared to be true for young female adults as well.[570] Normal urinary flow rates are perhaps slightly greater in females than males. Normal flow rates of 10 to 25 ml/sec have been suggested as a normal male range. Scott, Queseda and Cardus[453] recorded normal flow rates in men at 15.5 ml/sec to 16.2 ml/sec. Kauffman's[263] figures are somewhat higher, ranging from 13 to 26 and 20 to 44 ml/sec, as are Holm's[229] (20 to 30 ml/sec). The maximum voiding pressure in female children ranges between 30 to 60 cm of water, with a median value of 40 cm H_2O ($= 25$ mm Hg).[570] (The range here is applicable to male children, as well as to normal adults.)

Zinner, Ritter, Sterling and Harding[572] measured the flight distance of individual droplets of urine slightly distal to the vena contracta by high-speed cinematography, and were able to calculate the exit velocity of the urinary stream in their male subjects to be 150 to 250 cm/sec. Whitaker and Johnson[533] arrived at a calculated exit velocity of 398 cm/sec based upon direct pressure measurements with their tambour method.

It is probably impossible to establish an overall norm for these various pressure modalities, as there are marked individual variations in voiding patterns and pressures. Repeated measurements in a single patient have been reported to be more constant.[513]

The role of increased intra-abdominal pressure in urination has been adequately assessed.[180,465,512,513,514] It is now evident that increase in intra-abdominal pressure is not necessary for normal micturition. Voluntary fixation of the diaphragm and contraction of thoracic and abdominal musculature *do* increase the intravesical pressure but do not dramatically increase the flow rate[570,514,180] and, in fact, may reduce it to a certain extent. Enhorning[141] points out that the portion of the female urethra above the triangular ligament is also exposed to this increase in intra-abdominal pressure, and that in women with cystourethrocele it can be more of a hindrance than an aid to micturition.

The turbulence of urinary flow has only recently been considered a factor of importance.[355,335,336,570,464,465] Von Garrelts[514] has called attention to the most hydrodynamically favorable "funnel shape" of the vesical neck. Assuming that all urinary flow in both males and females is turbulent to some extent (rather than laminar), the degree of turbulence and consequent reduction in flow rate secondary to variations in the *shape* of the vesical neck and sphincteric urethra have yet to be adequately assessed. Rigid model studies[336,402] have shown that a rigid vesical neck lip with a dilated midurethral component is the least favorable conduit, and that a funnelled one, or one of uniform diameter throughout, is the most favorable (Fig. 34). Ritter, Zinner and Paquin[435] have called attention to the differences in shape of the urethral luminal contour during voiding; they regard it as a tube of numerous gullies and slits with a considerably smaller effective physiological diameter than one might imagine from measurements with a metal sound. Smith[464] has calculated the effective caliber of

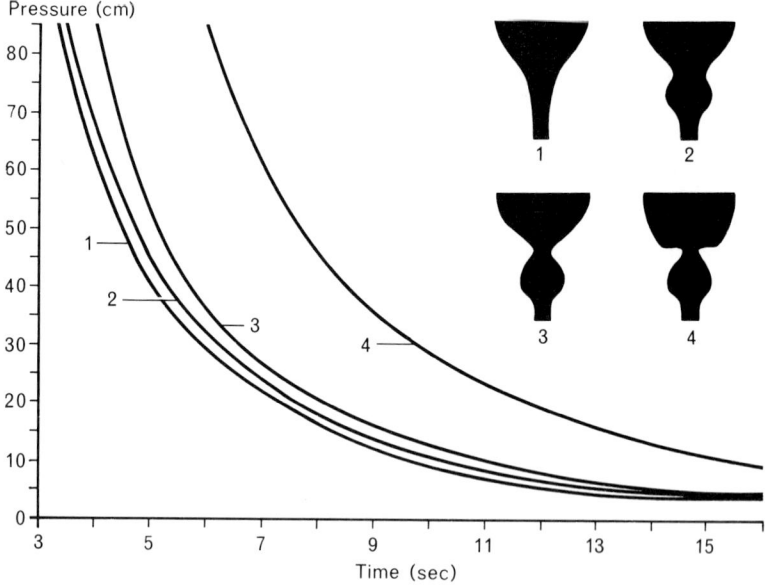

FIG. 34. Results of rigid model study showing relative flow rates of water through glass models of varying configuration. Luminal shapes were designed to simulate the vesical neck and sphincteric urethra. The most rapid flow was achieved with a funnelled form, or one of uniform caliber. (Courtesy of Professor H. Marberger, University of Innsbruck.)

the adult male urethra to be only 11 Fr (3.6 mm). The mucosal configuration, as well as that of the wall of the urethra, is responsible for turbulent flow. Consideration of underlying pathological processes which alter the optimal urethral configuration to produce reduced flow rates and possibly increased turbulence, resulting in even greater secondary structural damage from both pressure and infection, is of considerable importance.

To summarize the current state of our knowledge regarding the hydrodynamics of the lower urinary tract, it seems well established that increased urethral resistance is the primary cause of decreased flow and disturbed voiding patterns. The simple measurement of intravesical pressures alone is not sufficient evidence of outflow obstruction, due probably to the immense adaptability of the muscular components of the bladder. Voiding cystometry is not likely to be diagnostic in itself in marginally obstructing lesions of the sphincteric urethra.[119,570,182,183,515]

Ureteral reflux is not directly *due* to increased intravesical pressure in children.[62,570,236,4,5] This is probably also true in adult males, in whom acquired ureteral reflux in prostatic obstruction is uncommon,[358,357,61] and in paraplegics in whom associated atrophic neuromuscular derangement of the ureterovesical junction has been repeatedly demonstrated.[239,485] Neither is reflux directly related to lower urinary tract obstruction.[167] This tends to suggest that ureteral reflux is due to an abnormality of the ureterovesical junction.[474,242,319]

Resting pressures within the bladder are relatively constant for a single individual and show little change with increasing volumes (Mathieson). This simply confirms the fact that the detrusor adapts to its contents. Voiding pressure is relatively constant for a given individual, irrespective of the volume of contents within the bladder.

Intravesical pressure falls during urination, slowly with large volumes and more rapidly with small volumes. Von Garrelts[513,514] postulates that this is due to the shape of an excessively widened vesical neck and consequent decreased peripheral resistance.

Intravesical pressure rises some 5 to 6 seconds before urine starts to flow. Before the maximum voiding pressure is reached, urine appears at the urethral meatus. This confirms the anatomical structure of the smooth-muscle extensions and connections in the urethra, and stresses the importance of the bladder and sphincteric urethra as a single anatomical and functional unit.

Resting pressure within the bladder after urination is slightly lower than premicturition resting pressure.

Flow rate and urethral resistance are unrelated to decreasing mural tension in the detrusor wall during voiding in females. Urethral resistance does not differ significantly in female children with ureteral reflux and those without reflux.[570] Urinary flow rates were also found to be unchanged in a series of healthy young males voiding at altitudes of 36,000 feet.[93]

The voiding pattern (intermittency, prolongation, droplets, or even total inability to void) may indicate increased outflow resistance. Winter[550] has proposed the graphic representation of disturbed patterns by the use of radioisotope uroflowmetry. Auditory recordings of voiding patterns have been obtained.[327,267] Since disturbed voiding patterns in children can be due to many factors, their measurement should be regarded as a clinical observation and evaluated with caution.

The maximum urinary flow rate correlates very well with minimum urethral resistance and can be used clinically for this purpose.[570]

The ureterovesical junction functions normally as a one-way valve permitting entrance of urine into the bladder, but resisting its reflux. It is probably not breached by increased intravesical pressure alone, even in the newborn.[308]

The luminal diameter of the ureter varies from 0.1 to 0.5 mm and flow rates vary from 0 ml/min to 4 ml/min; peristaltic waves pass along it at a rate of 1 to 6 cm/sec. Peristaltic urinary flow within the ureter has a character of looping trajectories in which the central core of fluid moves generally downstream, but is surrounded by a sheath of fluid next to the ureteral wall moving generally upstream.[335,336]

IV
Pathology of Congenital Obstructive Lesions

Perhaps it has been wrong to think of sphincteric urethral obstruction as always a purely mechanical phenomenon, in the order of a cork or dam partially plugging the bladder outlet. At first glance, however, this is the most evident explanation. A large prostatic adenoma in an adult male obviously narrows the posterior urethra cystoscopically and radiographically. It is paradoxical, however, that elderly men with sometimes enormous lateral-lobe adenomatous hypertrophy have very few obstructive symptoms and no residual urine, while younger men with median bar formation or small middle-lobe (fibromyomatous) prostatic enlargement exhibit marked obstructive symptoms, hypertrophy of the detrusor and residual urine. Surgical removal of the obviously abnormal structures produces dramatic relief and seems to corroborate the impression of an offending plug of abnormal tissue as the cause of the obstruction.

We all understand the urological maxim that distal obstruction produces proximal dilatation and urinary stasis; this appears to be a basic urological truth. It is not surprising, therefore, that this concept has been transferred in its entirety to our thinking about lower urinary tract obstruction in infants and children.

Many descriptions have been published of obstructive abnormalities in children involving the vesical neck.[185,497,538,86,16,6,523,334, 284,426,143,307,54,434,214,65,516,351,77,219,2,85,9,109,153] Initially, this seemed to be a more or less straightforward problem of a conveniently obscure congenital nature, despite the fact that an actual plug or dam could not always be identified. The most widely held hypotheses suggested either hypertrophy of the smooth muscle of the vesical neck, submucosal fibrosis or fibroelastosis.

Many effective methods of treatment were then developed. The surgical reasoning supporting diagnosis and treatment, although in large measure excellent, has suffered the handicap of pragmatism. The main difficulty in management seemed to be that all available transurethral instruments were too large and that suprapubic exposure was inadequate.

In directly attacking the problem of what appeared to be obstruction at the neck of the bladder, Emmet and Hemholz[137] refined the transurethral approach. Burns,[66] Lich and Maurer[316, 317] and, subsequently, Hand and Sullivan,[207] Wilson, et al.,[547] Bonnin[30] and I[556] became early advocates of the retropubic approach for surgical attempts at correcting obstruction at the bladder neck or within the sphincteric urethra, as we seemed to find it. The retropubic exposure of the vesical neck and the performance of Y-V vesicourethroplasty in children with signs and symptoms of vesical-neck obstruction have been found to offer satisfactory relief in many cases,[557,559] despite the fact that we had no clear idea of the basic anomalies or their pathological appearance.

Information gained as a result of surgical intervention was then brought to bear upon the question of etiology. Although postoperative studies and results have been carefully analyzed by numerous authors,[194,304,381,332,333,97,544,67,430,466,266,191,51,10,212,376,68,342,505,443, 285,567,346,31,450] this has proven to be a less productive approach to the explanation of the underlying abnormality than one might suppose. In fact, the diversity of the obscure lesions producing such similar clinical findings appeared to challenge the entire mechanical concept.

It was assumed that Y-V vesicourethroplasty enlarged the vesical neck by turning it into a funnel, such as one observes after transurethral resection of the prostate. Alternately, it was considered possible that the rigidity and length of the supposed fibrotic bladder neck and sphincteric urethra were reduced by the insertion of the tongue of soft smooth muscle into the vesical neck.[377] Repeated biopsies taken from the vesical neck and posterior urethra, however, failed to reveal any predictable pathological changes.[560, 194, 74, 27]

It was evident that there was a sound neurological basis for a second type of apparent obstruction in some cases of dysraphism or obvious myelomeningocele, associated with myelodysplasia and spina bifida. The concomitant neurological deficits could be assessed and, despite the radiographic and endoscopic similarity to the idiopathic type of obstruction, this was clearly a neurogenic abnormality producing a functional neuromuscular imbalance of the detrusor-sphincter mechanism.[36, 168, 83, 136, 125, 104, 468] The response to surgery in these cases was unpredictable; although some cases have shown improvement, there have been few excellent results.

A third group of children with *no* evident pathology was soon recognized, and, although uncommon, the condition of megacystis began to be identified.[537, 538, 315, 391, 387] Here, there were some further differential diagnostic features: the widened trigone with laterally placed ureteral orifices and high incidence of ureteral reflux;[390] the cystometric findings of hypotonia of the detrusor; an increased bladder capacity; and the lack of signs indicating hypertrophy of the bladder musculature. Some observers believed that this syndrome was in some way related to an inability of the smooth muscle of the bladder wall itself to develop enough tone to balance even a surgically weakened vesical neck.

It has been postulated that this might be analogous to the aganglionic segments of bowel seen in Hirschsprung's disease [483, 484] or that it might represent an amyotonia on a cellular basis, either in the neuromuscular conduction system within the muscle bundles or within the smooth-muscle cell itself.[560] Smooth-muscle *dysplasia* can be demonstrated in cases of the "triad syndrome" of absent abdominal musculature, bilateral undescended testicles and urinary tract abnormality.[123, 234, 252, 385, 386, 459, 105] Here, again, surgical measures designed to relieve obstruction or, in these cases, to *balance* the detrusor and sphincter mechanism were unpredictable.[384, 543, 303]

A fourth and major differential diagnostic group of lesions in the sphincteric urethra, with a considerably better claim to obvious obstruction, has come under the general heading of *valves*. Mucosal folds and membranes, both above and below the verumontanum and within the bulbous and pendulous urethra, have been noted frequently.[541,272,143,425,426] Some appear to be definitely obstructing and some seem mere ridges on the posterior urethral wall.[475,388] In some reported cases[544,525,366,352,235,551] they are associated with apparent vesical-neck obstruction, and in others there seems to be no other obstructing lesion.[110,375,526] The diagnosis, both radiological and clinical, has been difficult and many times unsatisfying.

Radiographically and cystoscopically, there has frequently appeared to be a primary obstructive lesion in the bulbomembranous urethra of the male[92,331,305,415] and at the urethral meatus in the female,[326,327] so that there is a fifth contender for these diagnostic honors. The stimulus for this present inquiry has come from the paradoxical questions raised by attempts to separate these lesions both diagnostically and surgically.

It is important at this point to mention several other causes of infravesical obstruction occasionally accorded a place within this controversial family of lesions. Hypertrophy of the verumontanum has but rarely been described as a cause of urinary obstruction.[54,225,11,135] Congenital cysts of the prostatic urethra and vesical neck have been reported and successfully treated. Cystic and structural abnormalities of the wolffian and müllerian duct systems have been suspected, and in some cases proven to be primary lesions.[139,354,380,469] Polyps of the sphincteric urethra, also rare, can produce true mechanical obstruction.[120,542,504] Congenital urethral stricture of the cavernous urethra, anterior urethral valves,[524,231,84,306] and diverticula of the bulbous urethra related to developmental defects of the bulbo-urethral (Cowper's) ducts have also been noted[100,254,149,310] This group of miscellaneous lesions, however, stands somewhat apart from the primary five categories which have been characterized by their diagnostic obscurity and difficulty of treatment.

Taking the histotopographic view of the sphincteric urethra, it is evident that its function can be compromised not only by congenital lesions which (1) mechanically obstruct but also by those which (2) weaken the force of detrusor contraction, (3) produce imbalanced hypertrophy of the arcuate musculature, (4) produce rigidity of the sphincteric urethra, or (5) by inflammatory change lead to temporary edema and spasm of the delicate smooth-muscle balance between detrusor and sphincteric urethra. There are twelve clinically identifiable lesions which may exist as single entities, although frequently secondary functional changes in the sphincteric urethra supervene and may give the appearance of dual lesion, or at times even obscure the primary process.

Lesions of the Sphincteric and Distal Urethra
1. Valves
2. Fibrosis (fibroelastosis)
3. Vesical-neck hypertrophy
4. Urethral polyps
5. Urethral diverticulum
6. Cysts (Cowper's, müllerian)
7. Megacystis
8. Vesical dysplasia
9. Neurogenic bladder
10. Inflammatory lesions (urethritis, cystitis)
11. Urethral meatal stenosis
12. Tumor (rhabdomyosarcoma)

ETIOLOGY OF OBSTRUCTION

In this clinicopathological study, an attempt has been made to identify the various types of congenital urethral obstructions on an anatomical or embryological basis and to compare these findings with the normal histotopography of the infant urethra. Emphasis has been placed upon mural changes in the detrusor and sphincteric musculature, since its disturbed functions are direct reflections of disturbances in smooth-muscle integrity.

The pathological material includes four necropsy specimens with obstructive lesions from which 1,157 significant serial sections were obtained, and 60 biopsies from 33 surgical cases in children with various congenital obstructive lesions (see Tables 2 and 3 in *Introduction*, p. 4).

What are the underlying processes leading to the various lesions? Here, speculation and hypothesis must await ultimate molecular, maternal environmental, genetic and biochemical solutions.

Urethral Valves

In considering the origin and mode of obstruction of urethral valves, it may be well to consider an alternate hypothesis to the classical view of the three separate types of valves as conceived by

H. H. Young, Frontz and Baldwin.[563] This classical description, on purely clinical grounds, grouped together the inframontane cristal folds as type I valves, supramontane folds as type II valves, and diaphragmatic obstructions in the sphincteric urethra, both above and below the verumontanum, as type III valves. Based on anatomical studies of the sphincteric urethra and its embryological derivation, these three classic types have little in common. Robertson and Hayes[436] consider valvular obstruction to be diaphragmatic and *always* inframontane in their reported autopsy findings of 17 cases—one of the most carefully studied necropsy series in the literature.

Stephens, in 1963, reported his findings in a series of 47 cases, but may have been misled in his interpretation of the valve types by his method of dissection.

Robertson and Hayes, in "unroofing" the anterior (ventral) wall of the prostatic urethra, found the communication between the prostatic and distal urethra to consist merely of a small slit-like opening in a *diaphragm* across the lower portion of the prostatic urethra (Fig. 35). All of their diaphragms (rather than "valves," which they feel are artifactual due to a ventral splitting of the diaphragm during dissection) were located in the inframontane position. The diaphragm was found to be obliquely placed with its most cephalad point just beneath the verumontanum posteriorly, and its most caudal point within the membranous urethra anteriorly (ventrally).

Robertson and Hayes point out that the original Young, Frontz and Baldwin series of cases is open to obvious criticism: In the 12 reported cases there were only 5 postmortem examinations, of which one specimen was lost, another performed one year after operation, and in the other three it is unclear whether the autopsy examination was made by the authors or quoted from the autopsy report; in the remaining cases, classification was based only upon cystoscopic appraisal or operative findings.

The minute mucosal folds radiating caudally from the verumontanum as the plicae colliculi are notoriously difficult to evaluate cystoscopically, radiographically and anatomically. It is evident from the discussion of the superficial trigonal muscle that the supramontane folds frequently noted running from the vesical neck to the verumontanum are more related to the myoelastic superficial trigonal musculature than to the inframontane crista urethralis.

It is true that a few fibers of the superficial trigonal musculature

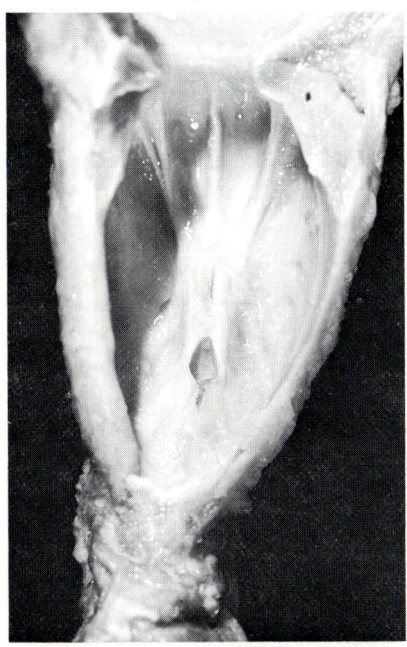

FIG. 35 Autopsy specimen of urethral diaphragm (valve). Ventral wall of prostatic urethra has been removed to reveal inframontane mucosal folds with central cavity. Note that the utricle (müllerian) is quite separate from this structure. The valve leaflets occupy the anatomical positions of the normal plicae colliculi. Prominent submucosal folds radiating upward from the verumontanum are unrelated and not obstructive. (Courtesy of Robertson and Hayes.)

bifurcate around the verumontanum and continue into the inframontane urethra along its dorsal surface as the prostatourethral fibers, ending their course in the membranous urethra. The inframontane crista urethralis (or plicae colliculi), however, has a different structure and a more superficial submucosal distribution than these prostatourethral fibers, and it is proposed that the embryological origin of the inferior cristal folds is different from that of the superficial trigonal muscle: specifically, that they arise from the original urethrovaginal (ventrolateral[60,279]) folds of the urogenital sinus which, in the female, form the anterior half of the hymenal ring and, in the male, remain as plical vestiges with radial insertions into the bulbous urethra distal to the meatus of Guyon. These folds represent, in their various manifestations, urethral valves (Fig. 36).

G. S. Thompson[498] likened these inframontane valvular folds to an "imperforate hymen." There are also Lowsley's[322] description of cristal fibers attaching themselves around the circumference of the urethra and Watson's case[527] in which the verumontanum was assumed to be adherent to the roof (i.e., ventral wall) of the urethra. Knox and Sprunt[274] noted circumferential attachment and adherence anteriorly of valve leaflets, in which case there was a *posterior slit* communicating with the urethra. The case of Fuchs[163] quoted by them showed a "vaginal cavity" *behind* the valves.

Tolmaltschew[500] reported one case with an enlarged "utriculus," and Young, Frontz and Baldwin[563] noted one case with a dilated "sinus pocularis."

This is consonant with the embryological origin of the urethrovaginal folds, as initially in the pelvic urogenital sinus they are attached anterolaterally in the 40-mm embryo to form the "crista-urethralis anterior."[60] The fact that the inframontane cristal folds are double and, in cases of valves, ordinarily symmetrical, calls for an embryological origin from a bifid structure within the pelvic urogenital sinus. Wolffian and müllerian structures, in order to produce an anomaly with the prime characteristic of duplication, can reasonably be held responsible only for duplicated anomalies *above* the verumontanum.

Anomalous development of the wolffian and müllerian ducts (Lowsley[322] and Stephens[475]) was proposed as the defect responsible for valve formation on the basis that the wolffian ducts opened "close to" the cloacal membrane in the 4-mm fetus. This latter view would seem to be untenable in that the inframontane folds radiate caudally and ventrally from the verumontanum (the original müllerian hillock). Since the müllerian ducts develop within the sheath of the wolffian ducts and open together with them at the verumontanum (Gruenwald[195]), it seems most unlikely that mucosal folds distal to the müllerian hillock on the dorsal surface of the urethra could be related in any way to either of these duct systems. Then, the question is: What paired primordial structures exist in the wall of the pelvic

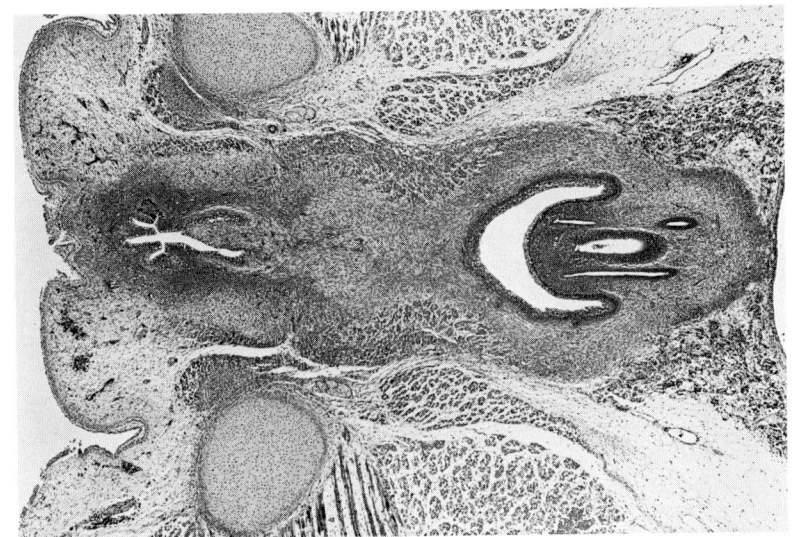

A

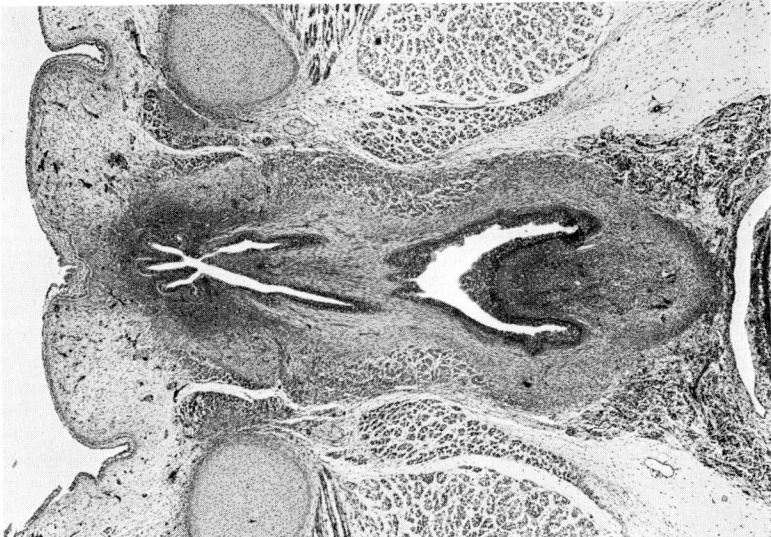

B

FIG. 36. Selected serial coronal sections progressing from ventral to dorsal aspects of the inframontane urethra in a 55-mm human embryo. The fused müllerian ducts (utricle) occupy the center of the verumontanum at right in *A*. Note symmetrical ejaculatory ducts (wolffian) in close proximity. Primitive musculature of sphincteric urethra is evident at this stage. Stellate cavity at left represents developing bulbomembranous urethra (pars pelvina of urogenital sinus).

Opening of Cowper's ducts into the bulbous urethra can be seen in *B* (at left). Section slightly more dorsal.

Section through base of the verumontanum (right). Prominent declevities to either side would be analogous to "sinus bays" in the female.

C

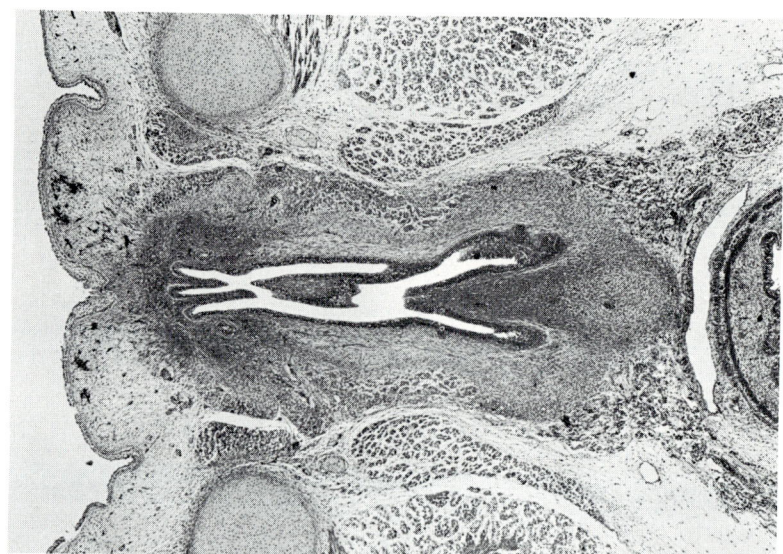

D

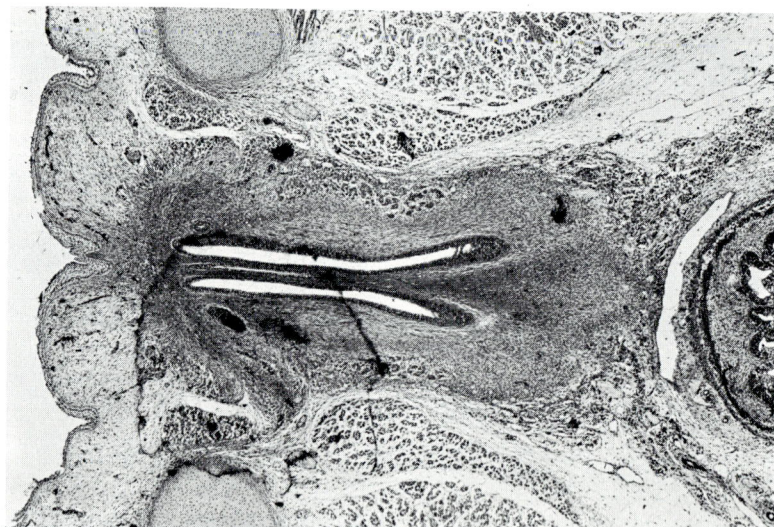

FIG. 36. Note attachment of regressing urethrovaginal fold to ventrolateral wall of urethra center. Cowper's ducts and bulbous urethra in C at left.

Plical folds extending from the verumontanum to region of future bulbous urethra in D. Note central cleft.

Compare with diaphragmatic orifice and valve leaflets in case of Robertson and Hayes (Fig. 35), and with Unterkircher anomaly (Figs. 41B and 43).

portion of the urogenital sinus proper which could account for dorsal urethral mucosal folds in the male only? The anomalies in this region related to the formation of the urogenital sinus portion of the vagina point directly to a disturbance in the regression of the urethrovaginal folds (anterior hymenal anlage) as the embryological basis for inframontane valve formation.

Supramontane *diaphragmatic* obstructions, as reported rarely in the literature, are difficult if not impossible to explain embryologically, and future cases must be carefully studied in serial section in order to place them. With this reservation in mind, it is proposed that the term "valve" *be reserved for abnormalities of the crista urethralis (plicae colliculi)* and be limited to the inframontane urethra. This probably includes cases reported as *hypertrophy* of the verumontanum, in which cristal folds were noted inserting into the walls or roof of the inframontane urethra and perhaps accounts, in large measure, for the tethered obstruction in the bulbomembranous urethra due to the radial insertion of normal-appearing cristal folds at this point.

It is not inconceivable that a defect in the regression of the original urethrovaginal folds can be influenced by genetic fault or prenatal hormonal changes in the fetus or mother.[217, 108] Reul and Ansell[431] report one instance of an urethral valve in one monozygotic twin; the other was found to have bulbomembranous stenosis. The mother had continued to take a progesterone preparation by mouth for part of her first trimester, unaware that she was pregnant. Varying degrees of persistence—from completely obstructing, large, sail-like, bifid valves at one end of the scale to barely visible, distal, bifurcated plicae colliculi at the other—are perhaps all variations in this same regressive process (Fig. 37). This view agrees with the clinical observations that the type I valve is the most common, and that resection or excision of the inframontane cristal folds produces relief of the valvular obstruction. The type III diaphragmatic valve in the inframontane position is probably only a variation of this embryological abnormality. Type II valves do not exist as separate entities. They are merely accentuations of the hypertrophied superficial trigonal muscle and are never primarily obstructing.

It is of further significance that true urethral valves have not been reported in the female and, although Nesbit, McDonald and Busby[379] were able to demonstrate redundant mucosal folds in the female urethra, these cannot be embryologically related to the genesis of the

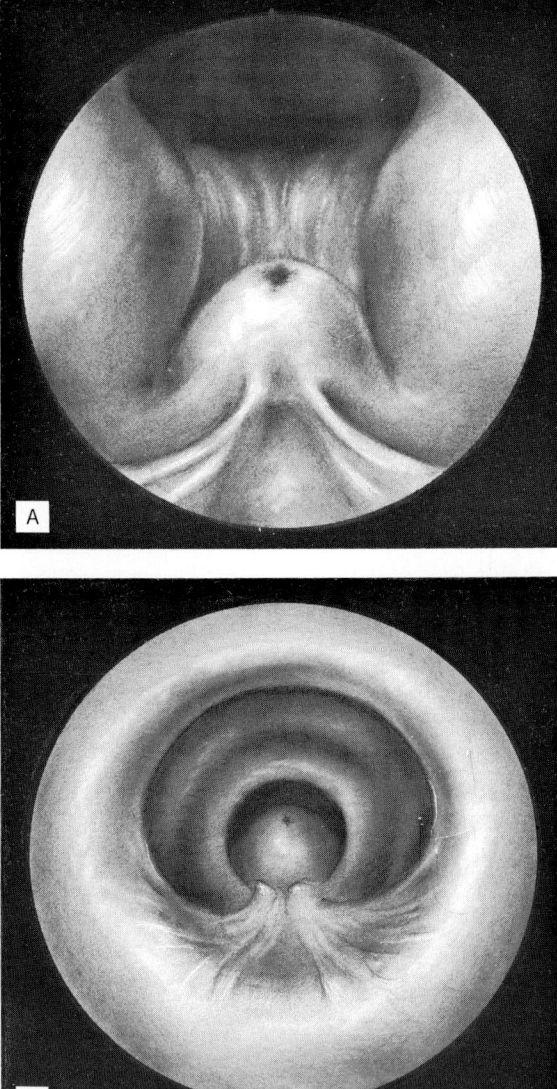

FIG. 37. Drawings of the cystoscopic appearance of excessively prominent inframontane plicae colliculi arising from the base of the verumontanum (*A*).

In *B*, the panendoscope has been withdrawn into the bulbous urethra. The plical folds (valves) can be seen extending through the distal limit of the external sphincter (meatus of Guyon). The splayed bulbomembranous insertions of the tethering valvular folds produce annular stenosis at this point.

male inframontane valves unless they are considered as part of the confluent hymenal component of the dorsal urethral meatus.

It has been noted that the inframontane crista urethralis (plicae colliculi) is always absent in cases of valvular urethral obstruction. Voiding cystourethrography in the male is further consonant with this view, in that the arrest of urine during micturition rarely occurs at the site of the oblique valvular markings within the sphincteric urethra but ordinarily at a site near their distal limits, and is of a circular or arcuate nature (Fig. 38). The proximal dilatation of the sphincteric urethra, particularly anteriorly, and the accentuation of the trigonal and detrusor loops representing the vesical neck cannot reasonably be considered to be primarily obstructive.

Bulmer's[58,59,60] observations in humans and sheep indicate that the anterior and posterior portions of the hymen are formed differently. The anterior portion is derived from the ventrolateral folds in the urogenital sinus wall at the level of the caudal outpouching of the dorsolateral wings of sinus epithelium which mark the future orifice of the vagina. These urethrovaginal folds, one on each side (extending distally to the bulbo-urethral glands), are the anterior paired segments of the hymen.

The posterior, unpaired segment of the hymen develops by a type of accordion pleating of the dorsal wall of the urogenital sinus as the vagina increases in size. In this view, the hymen is derived entirely from the urogenital sinus caudal to the müllerian tubercle.

In order to confirm this hypothetical origin of urethral valves, one should ideally be able to examine several anomalous embryos at various stages of development—or, at least, be fortunate enough to stumble upon a single fetus with such an anomaly. Such a fortuitous occurrence is dramatically demonstrated in the studies of the case reported here, in which symmetrical, sail-like valves obstructing the inframontane urethra were present in association with a more distal atresia of the urethra. The study of this case is particularly interesting in that it provides embryological evidence for two different sites of obstruction. The valvular obstruction in this case was 9 mm proximal to the atresia of the urethra and the urethral atresia was associated with total failure of the cloacal membrane. This points clearly to a difference between the site of urogenital membrane obstruction and that of valvular obstruction. Evidence in these studies has shown that the structure of the serially sectioned valve and the structure of the

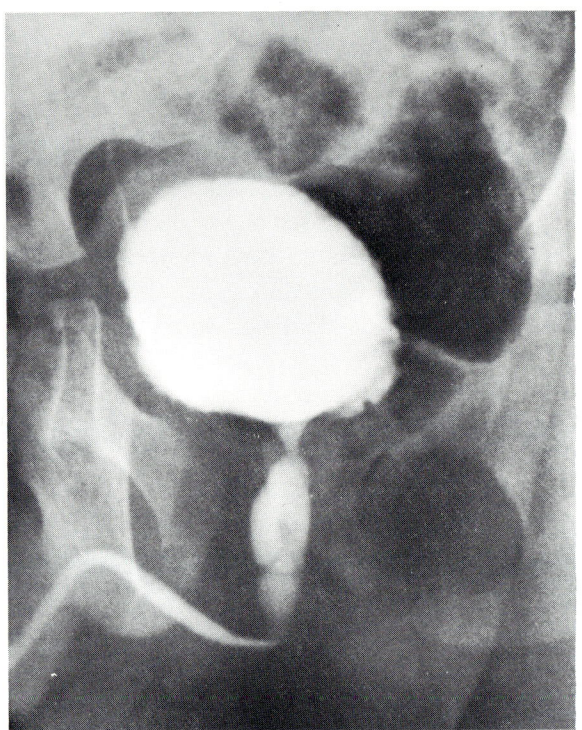

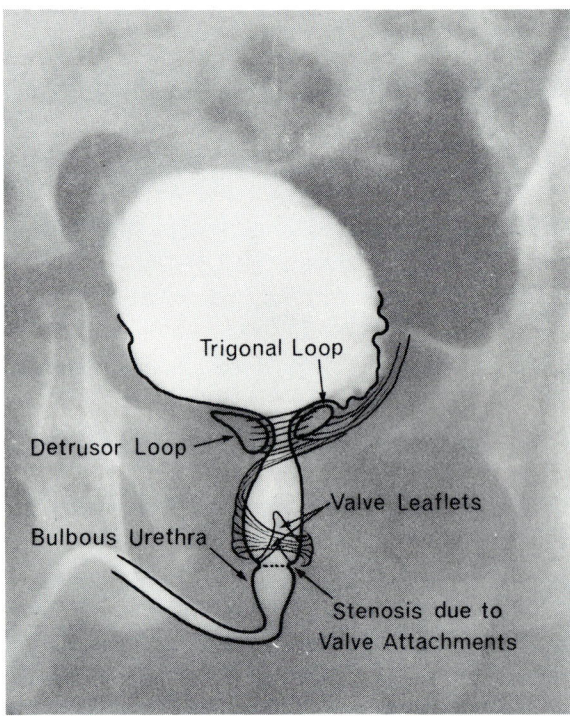

FIG. 38. Oblique voiding cystourethrogram in 7-year-old boy with urethral valvular obstruction. Note annular site of obstruction at distal insertions of valvular folds. Hypertrophy of detrusor (including the vesical neck) and trabeculation are secondary changes.

normal hymenal ring are almost identical, having merely a superior and inferior epithelial covering with a collagen and elastic fiber core. Only rare smooth-muscle cells were noted in the entire series of the valve sections.

Valves in the anterior urethra are unrelated to this embryological defect, though they may well represent faulty fusion of the phallic portion of the urogenital sinus in formation of the urethra.

THE UNTERKIRCHER ANOMALY

One bright, snowy day in February of 1966, in the laboratory of the Anatomy and Embryology Institute of the University of Innsbruck, Doctor Konrad Unterkircher and I dissected a 48-cm stillborn infant which had been sent to the Institute from the hospital in Zams with the sole explanation that it was a case of atresia ani and possible intersex (Fig. 39).

A full description of the gross anatomy of Doctor Unterkircher's

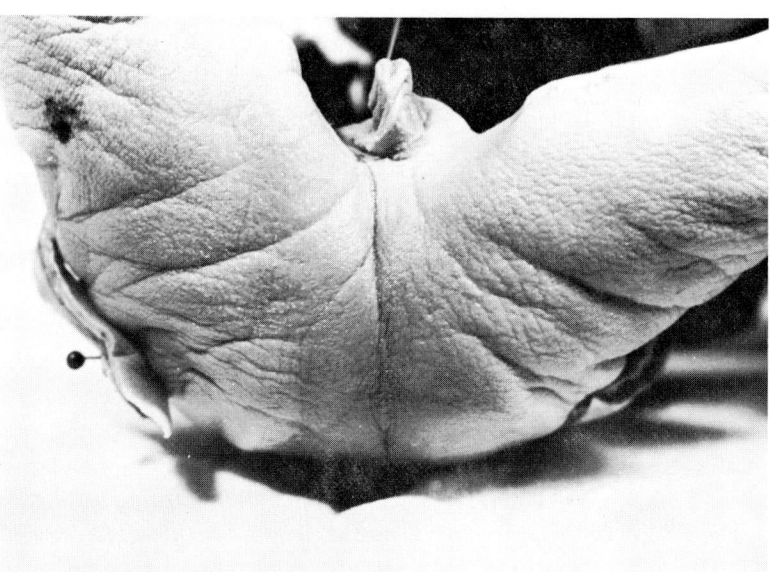

FIG. 39. Unterkircher anomaly. Photograph of the perineum of stillborn, formalin preserved, male infant with imperforate anus and aplasia of the penis. Multiple urogenital anomalies are present.

anomaly will be only abstracted here. This was a term, male infant preserved in formalin, 48 cm in crown-heel length. Anomalies in the specimen included inperforate anus with congenital rectovesical fistula, absent right kidney, dysplastic cystic left kidney, aplasia of the penis, aplasia of the urethra and corpora cavernosa, intra-abdominal testes with normal vasa deferentia and epididymides, a partial "urogenital sinus vagina," and the presence of urethral valves at a site different from the aplastic occlusion of the urethra. Chromosomal karyotyping could obviously not be carried out. The sex chromatin was male.

In the open abdominal cavity, the distended bladder had the appearance of two ovoid cavities: one lying in the craniocaudal plane and extending obliquely toward the anterior abdominal wall, and a second communicating freely with it and attached to the umbilicus via the urachus (Fig. 40). The distal portion of the specimen connected with the inferior cavity and terminated in a funnelled neck corresponding roughly to the inframontane urethra. At its most distal end it was occluded, and connected only by a thin fibrous band to the atretic bulbous urethra. There was no anus. The rectum communicated with the superior portion of the hugely dilated, inferior ovoid cavity at a point approximately 1 cm medial to the entrance of both vasa deferentia. The ureter draining the solitary dysplastic kidney opened slightly cephalad and posterior to the rectovesical communication. The bladder, dysplastic kidney, connection of the rectum with the prostatic urethra and the bulbous urethra were excised carefully en bloc.

When the specimen was opened through its ventral surface with an incision bisecting the urachus, the upper ovoid cavity was found to represent the bladder proper. The constriction between the two cavities represented the bladder neck, and the inferior (larger of the two cavities) represented the entire sphincteric urethra. Both cavities showed heavy trabeculation; the mucosa was shiny and clear throughout. As the incision was continued through the region of the assumed membranous urethra from the ventral aspect, a perfect bicuspid urethral valve was identified. Distal to the most inferior limit of this valve, which arose from the anterolateral walls of the urethra, was a triangular cavity measuring 9 mm in length. At the distal end of this cavity the atretic bulbomembranous urethra was encountered (Figs. 41*A, B*). Each valve leaflet measured 4 mm in width from the midline to its anterolateral connection with the urethral wall. The cephalocaudal extent of the valves, measured from the midline base,

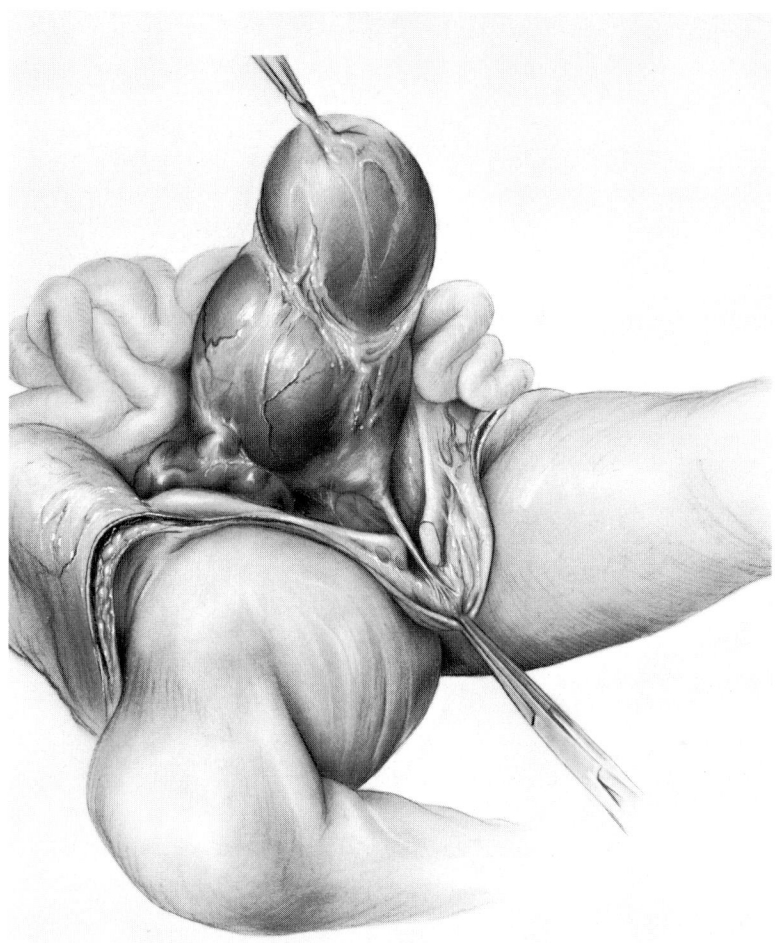

FIG. 40. Unterkircher anomaly. Drawing of the gross appearance of the opened abdominal cavity. The distorted bladder consists of two communicating ovoid cavities. The atretic urethra ends blindly in the loose pudendal skin. The solitary cystic dysplastic kidney can be seen within the bony pelvis at left.

was 7 mm. A slight bulge at the base of the valves had the appearance of the müllerian tubercle; however, it was found to be composed only of a collagenous and elastic core with epithelial linings on both sides of the same transitional structure as that composing the valves. The length of this region was 3 mm.

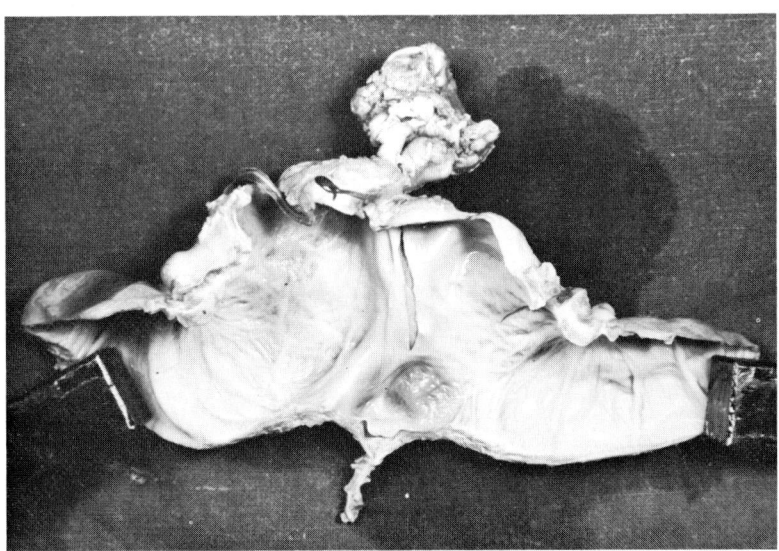

FIG. 41. *A*, Unterkircher anomaly. Photograph of opened bladder and sphincteric urethra. Dysplastic kidney remains attached to the upper portion of the specimen. Note valvular folds (bottom center) and opened retrourethral cavity. One of the vasa deferentia is visible at upper left.

Beneath the valvular structures a probe could be inserted through a narrowed area and then passed the entire length of the sphincteric urethra along a tubular cavity arising *beneath* the urethral valves. The length of the cavity was 7.5 cm. It was 13 mm wide, uniformly, except for the constriction at the base of the urethral valves, which measured 3 mm. The width of the membranous urethra at its widest point (the connection of the urethral valves to the lateral wall) measured 1.4 cm.

At a point 1.5 cm distal to the completely atretic portion of the bulbous urethra, a careful transverse incision revealed a tiny dysplastic urethral lumen less than 1 mm in diameter. 723 serial and step microscopic sections were made of the entire atretic, bulbous, membranous and posterior walls of the sphincteric urethra to the entrance of the vasa deferentia and ureter.

Microscopically, the atretic urethra was represented by a tiny lumen with a transitional cell mucosa (Fig. 42), surrounded by a dense layer of collagen. There was no evidence of smooth muscle, elastic tissue or striated muscle and no evidence of corpus spongiosum sur-

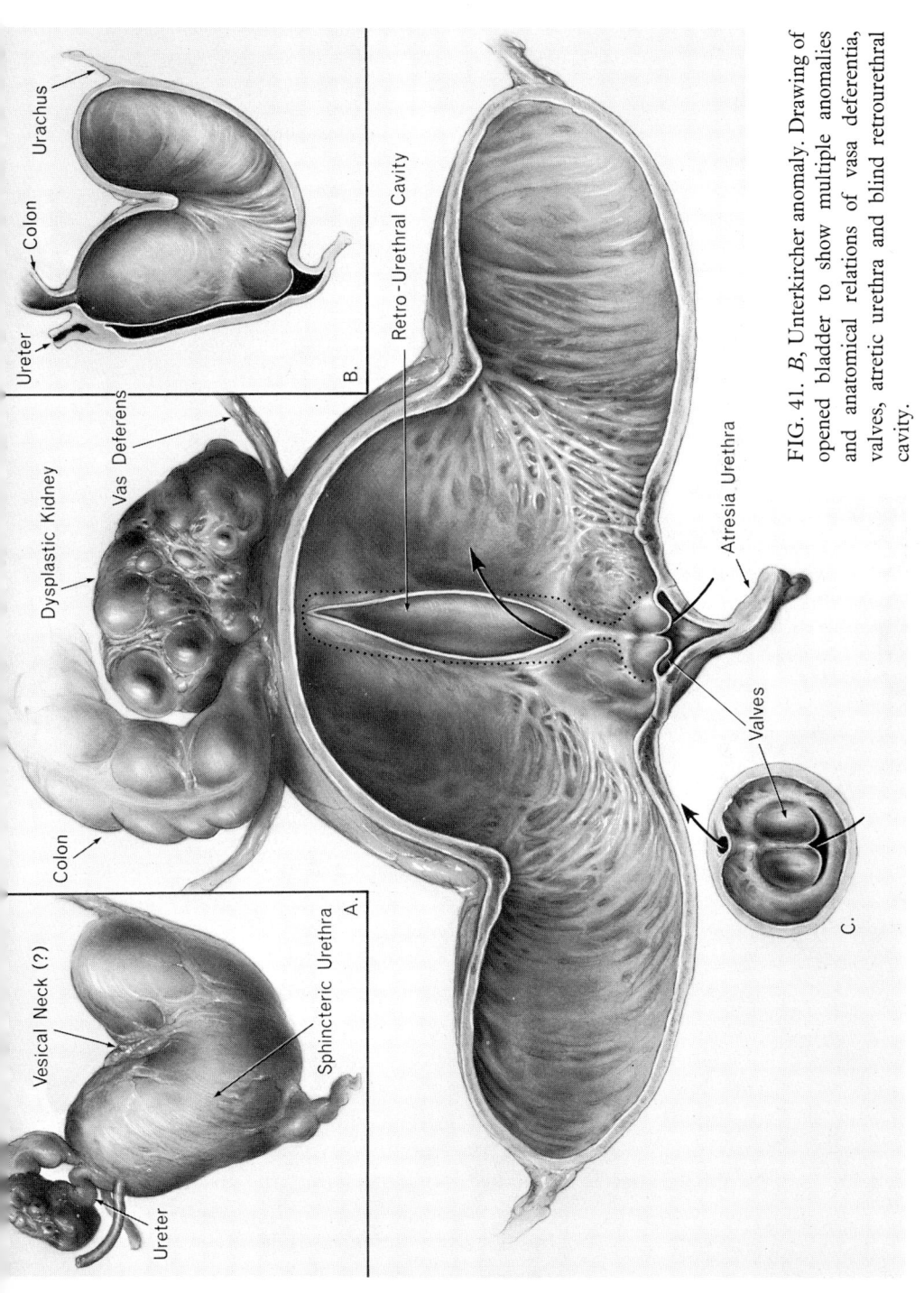

FIG. 41. *B*, Unterkircher anomaly. Drawing of opened bladder to show multiple anomalies and anatomical relations of vasa deferentia, valves, atretic urethra and blind retrourethral cavity.

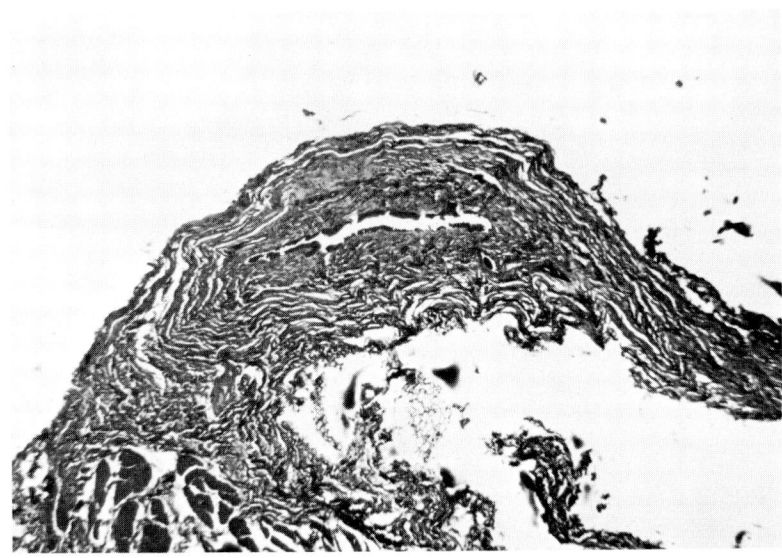

FIG. 42. Photomicrograph of transverse section through atretic portion of urethra. Lumen was less than 1 mm in diameter. Trichrome stain, Goldner modification. Original magnification X30.

rounding the urethra. The submucosa showed many short collagen fibers with a disorganized pattern. One small urethral gland was noted.

The valve leaflet surrounding the sphincteric urethra sectioned transversely showed the leaflets to be composed entirely of collagen and fine elastic fibers (Fig. 43). A few well differentiated blood vessels were noted. There were only isolated smooth-muscle cells. The membranous urethra in this region was lined with sparse transitional epithelium. A loose tunica propria was composed almost entirely of collagen. There was no submucosal layer of elastic tissue to be seen, unlike the normal membranous urethra, particularly in its dorsal aspect, where one would expect to see large, dense layers of elastic tissue representing the crista urethralis. Longitudinal smooth muscle was found immediately beneath the tunica propria; some bundles were cut obliquely and circular smooth muscles were found in the next superficial layer. There was marked fibroelastosis in these layers. Superficial to this were a few longitudinal smooth-muscle bundles. Peripheral muscle distributed in a circular pattern beneath the longitudinal smooth muscle of the adventitia showed striations and probably represented the "intrinsic striated" urethral sphincter. Longitudinal

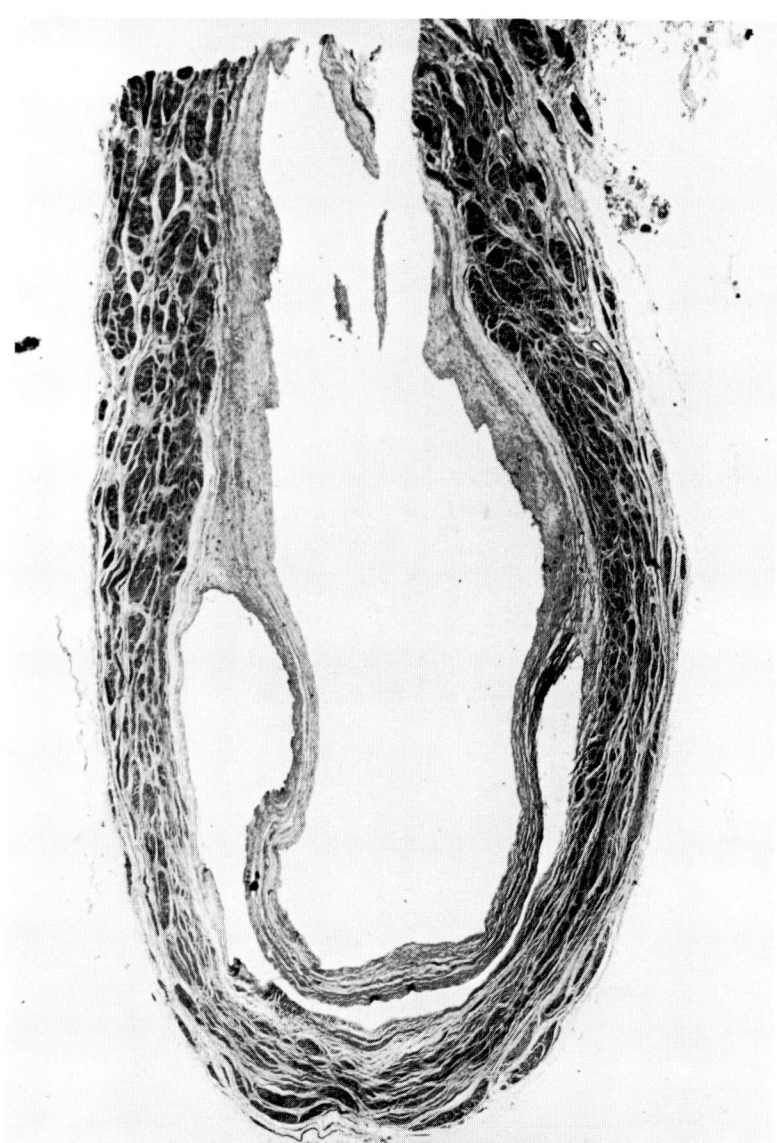

FIG. 43. Unterkircher anomaly. Photomicrograph of section through conjoined valve leaflets. Muscle bundles of urethral wall are darkly stained. There are no muscle cells within the valve leaflets. Note the similarity of lateral origins of leaflets to the normal mural attachments of the developing plicae colliculi in Fig. 36C. Trichrome stain, Goldner modification. Original magnification X15.

smooth-muscle fibers overlying this could be considered to be vesico-prostatourethral fibers.

Sections through the midportion of the posterior wall of the sphincteric urethra showed the sinus cavity to be composed of collagenous fibers entirely (Fig. 44). There were no elastic fibers and no smooth-muscle cells. The cavity was lined on both sides by a transitional epithelium. Immediately beneath the mucosa was a loose tunica propria continuous with that forming the core of the anterior (ventral) wall of the "urogenital sinus vagina." Beneath the tunica propria there were a few longitudinal smooth-muscle bundles. A "midcircular layer" showed some of the bundles cut obliquely. To the right side of the specimen was a muscular ridge with finer smooth-muscle bundles cut longitudinally. This ridge had been previously noted in the gross dissection and extended cranially to the base of the "urogenital sinus vagina," increasing in thickness. No lumen or epithelial structures could be identified. There were no squamous

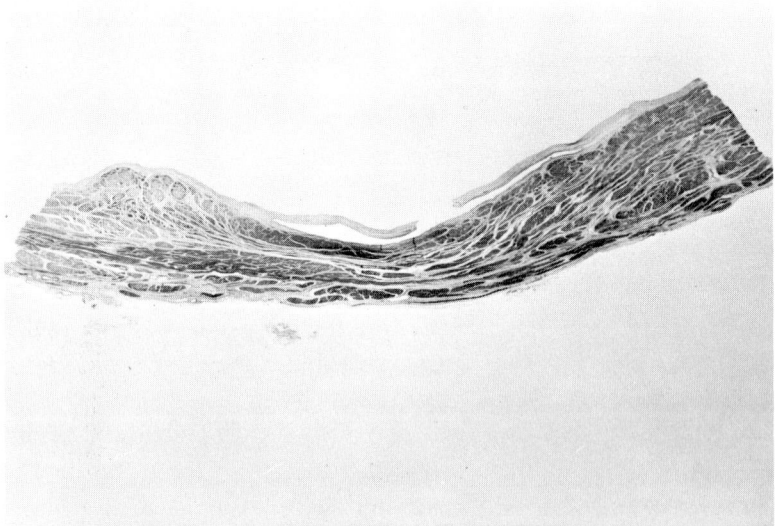

FIG. 44. Unterkircher anomaly. Transverse section through midportion of retrourethral cavity. Muscle bundles in sphincteric urethra are distorted and show marked fibroelastosis. The opened cavity shows the same collagen core as the valve leaflets distal to it.

changes in the epithelium to suggest estrogen influence. No goblet cells or rectal mucosa were found in any section. No prostatic acini or seminal vesicles were visible in any of the sections.

In consideration of the Unterkircher anomaly, one of the most significant problems is the orientation of the cavity arising behind the valve leaflets. In an effort to localize the site of the atresia of the urethra and valve cusps, the criteria available are: (1) Pennington's elastic arc, (2) smooth-muscle distribution of the sphincteric urethra, (3) striated-muscle distribution, (4) nerve and ganglion distribution, (5) prostatic ducts, (6) müllerian elements, (7) site of entry of vasa deferentia and site of entry of the ureter, (8) estrogen-influenced epithelium of the urogenital sinus, and (9) identification of a bulbo-urethral gland and duct system (Cowper's—Bartholin's).

The fact that in this specimen both vasa deferentia were present and attached to normal testes with epididymides indicates the presence of both wolffian ducts and mesonephros. The unilateral kidney could suggest either the failure of ureteral budding from the left wolffian duct or the failure of metanephrogenic blastema development on this side. The site of entrance of the vasa deferentia at the most cranial extent of the cavity established this as the original site of the müllerian hillock (genital cord) at which the original mesonephric and müllerian ducts would have opened (if Gyllensten's[199] assumptions are correct). This effectively rules out the caudal cavity as being a müllerian duct cyst and indicates its origin from the urogenital sinus.

The association of dysplastic stenosis of the urethra with an imperforate anus, absence of the penis and lack of a phallic opening of the urogenital sinus would indicate the site of the urethral atresia at the cloacal membrane, of which, in this specimen, there was apparently almost complete failure.

The most likely analogy, in view of these findings, is that the cavity arising behind the valve leaflets represented the urogenital sinus portion of the vagina. The fact that the site of valvular attachment to the vault of the abortive sphincteric urethra was clearly proximal by 9 mm and separate from the area of atresia points to *two entirely different sites of obstruction*: the more distal atretic one related to failure of the cloacal membrane, and the valvular formation due to persistence of the urethrovaginal folds of the pelvic urogenital sinus with the confirmatory presence of the posteriorly placed vaginal cavity ending blindly at the müllerian hillock.

Fibroelastosis

The clinical identification of vesical-neck obstruction in childhood has preceded its pathological identification by many years. The difficulties with diagnosis and variable response to surgery have made it obvious that primary idiopathic vesical-neck contracture, although dignified as a syndrome, has been often incriminated as the offending lesion when associated with any of the obstructive lesions of the sphincteric urethra.

Campbell[74] identified submucous fibrosis histologically in many of his cases. Bodian[27] in 1957 described the histology of the posterior urethra in five cases of idiopathic bladder-neck obstruction in infants who came to autopsy. He felt that the primary lesion was fibroelastosis of an abnormally elongated urethra. He noted, particularly, an increased prominence of elastic fibers below the level of the verumontanum. His controls and a single case of posterior urethral valves failed to show this quantitative difference in elastic tissue. Others have reported biopsies of the vesical neck to show hypertrophy of smooth muscle, fibrosis and chronic inflammation. Gross, Randolph and Wise[194] found no consistent histological pattern in 22 of their cases of Y-V plasty in which biopsies were obtained. My own cases[556,557,559,560] have shown no predictable histological changes.

There does appear to be a group of children with definite constriction of the vesical neck, hypertrophied detrusor musculature with cellules and diverticula, and often with severe upper-tract dilatation, who show no other obstructive lesion in the sphincteric or distal urethra. Moreover, there is good reason to believe that this particular lesion is familial. Keitzer and Benavent[266] found that, in their 303 children with bladder-neck obstruction who required vesical-neck surgery, one or more of their siblings and the father or mother exhibited similar lesions in varying degrees. This association was present in 66 of the families of their patients. Of these familial obstructions, 122 cases were considered mild, 145 cases showed moderate obstruction, but 36 cases showed advanced obstruction with hydronephrosis and infection. Though no histological findings were reported, these authors suggested that the lesion causing increased resistance involved the entire sphincteric urethra in both male and female.

Finkle, McPhee and Van der Reis[148] reported pure contracture of the vesical neck in two male American Indian-Caucasian brothers, age $5\frac{1}{2}$ and $6\frac{1}{2}$, with severe upper-tract damage.

In one of my cases reported by Young and Goebel in 1954,[557] Y-V plasty for vesical-neck obstruction (with no distal associated lesion) producing severe upper-tract dilatation was carried out. The patient had an excellent long-term result, had no further difficulties with urination or ejaculation, was subsequently married, and his first son was found to have an identical lesion of the vesical neck with marked obstructive changes. Y-V vesicourethroplasty was subsequently carried out in the son by Dr. James Goebel and Dr. John Hutch (Figs. 45*A*, *B* and *C*). One of my patients, a 45-year old woman with classical vesical-neck contracture and a histological picture of fibroelastosis in the biopsy specimen, had an excellent result from Y-V vesicourethroplasty, as had a younger brother some years previously for an apparently congenital contracture of the vesical neck.

In eight cases of carefully selected idiopathic congenital vesical-neck obstruction, four of whom were female and four male,[560] dense fibroelastosis of the vesical neck was the principal histological finding (Fig. 46). The elastic fibers in general occupied the intermuscular septa and the elastic fibers in these areas were of the heavy, discrete type; they were not arranged in any particular layer, but aligned with the smooth-muscle bundles and roughly parallel to the collagenous elements in the vesical neck and urethra. There was no increase in the elastic fibers of the tunica propria. In fact, elastic fibers were as uncommon as in the normal controls. In two of the adult males, there was an increase in the collagen of the tunica propria.

The clinical criteria for this diagnosis must include a life-long history of an obstructed voiding pattern and hypertrophy of the detrusor, with the usual finding of severe upper urinary tract involvement. The demonstration on voiding cystourethrography of definite obstruction *only* at the vesical neck is of major importance. Biopsy of the vesical-neck musculature and midurethral segment should show histological evidence of definite fibroelastosis. In addition, a careful history may include a sibling or parent who, when studied, will reveal the same abnormality.

It is extraordinarily difficult to indict primary fibroelastosis as the principal lesion in these cases; the most marked general response of the bladder musculature to aging, neurological dysfunction, overstretching, interstitial cystitis and even hypertrophy is a deposition of large amounts of elastin between muscle bundles. Elastin is seen in association with intact muscle fascicles in detrusor hypertrophy and is noted as a replacement for dysplastic, degenerated or sheared

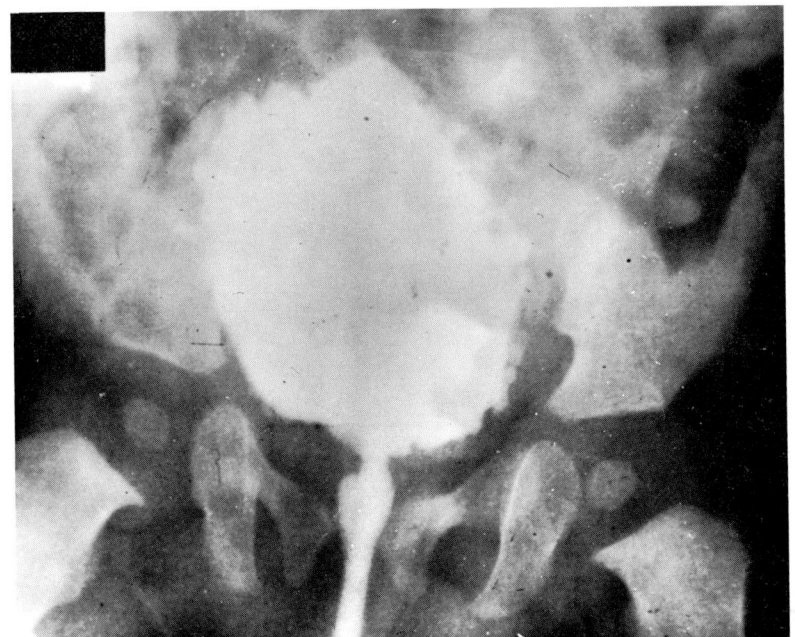

A

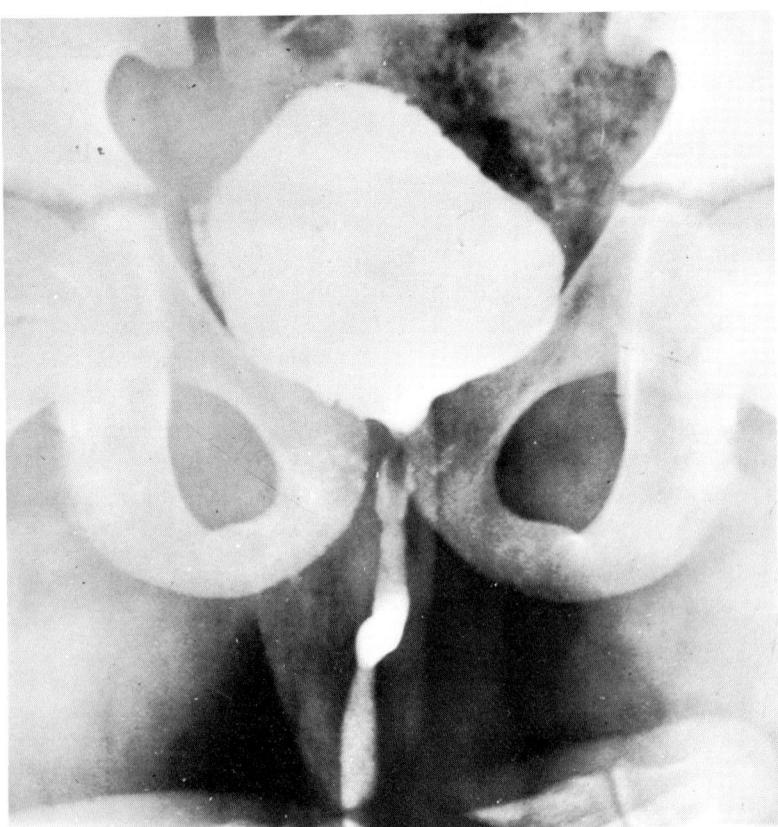

B

FIG. 45. *See legend on facing page.*

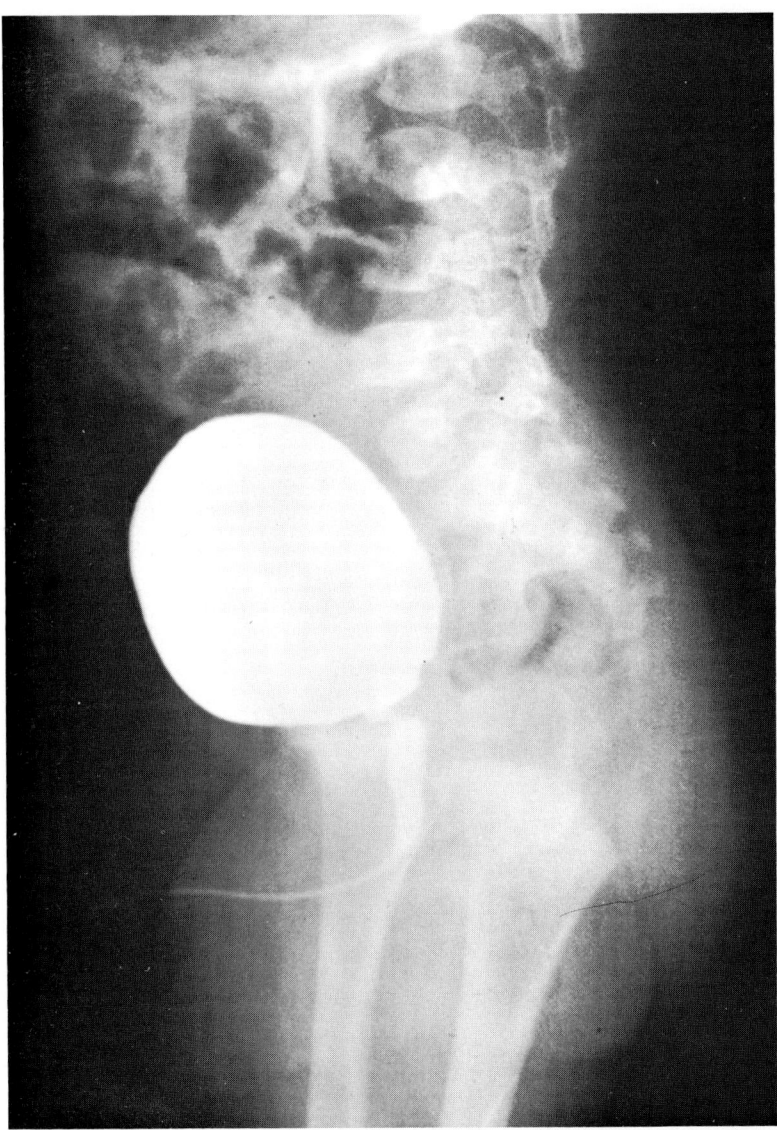

C

FIG. 45. Retrograde cystourethrogram in a male infant made in 1954 with history of repeated episodes of urinary retention from the age of 2 days (A). Note heavily trabeculated bladder. The sphincteric urethra is poorly seen due to the inlying catheter. Y-V vesicourethroplasty was carried out. Postoperative voiding cystourethrogram at the age of 11 years shows widely funnelled vesical neck extending almost to the verumontanum (B). Voiding cystourethrogram of the patient's son (C) taken in 1966 showing pure vesical neck obstruction.

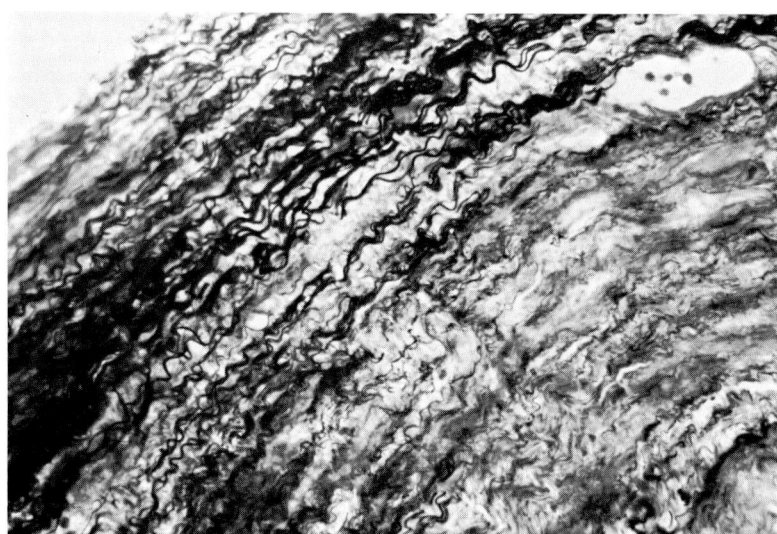

FIG. 46. Photomicrograph of biopsy specimen from the vesical neck of a 6-year-old boy removed at the time of Y-V vesicourethroplasty. Smooth-muscle fascicles and some individual cells are interlaced with elastic fibers (black) at lower right. Collagen and abnormally thickened elastic fibers almost completely replace the smooth muscle at upper left. Verhoeff-van Gieson stain. Original magnification X400.

smooth-muscle fascicles (Fig. 47). Elastosis is conspicuously absent from the tunica propria and is quite unlike the fibroelastosis occurring in the hearts of newborns with severe congenital heart disease.

The histological character of the elastic fiber noted in fibroelastosis is more that of pseudoelastin[203,122,204,205] and bears little resemblance to the normal elastic layers noted in the inframontane and membranous urethra of the male. Bodian's description of elastotic change throughout the sphincteric urethra in his cases may be explained by elastosis involving all of the musculature of the sphincteric urethra. It is, of course, possible that this histological picture is an entirely secondary phenomenon, even though present at birth. The underlying stimulus for this fibroelastosis must remain speculative at present.

Vesical-Neck Hypertrophy

Marion[338] attributed bladder neck obstruction in children to hypertrophy of the smooth-muscle bundles of the internal sphincter at the vesical neck and, without the additional aids of voiding cinecystourethrography and the current knowledge of hydrodynamics of the urinary tract, this appeared to be an attractive explanation.

It has been pointed out by numerous authors[458,526,335,318,271] that although apparent prominence of the vesical neck can exist, particularly in relation to a dilated distal sphincteric urethra, the actual caliber is not reduced and the obstructive phenomena occurring at an hypertrophied vesical neck are more related to (1) the inability of the longitudinal musculature of the bladder to draw the hypertrophied arcuate loops away from the vesical neck, and (2) a reduction in flow due to exaggerated turbulence produced by the vesical-neck deformity.[336] Varying degrees of prominence of the vesical neck occur in association with valvular or membranous stenosis, strictures of the bulbous urethra, and neurogenic dysfunction secondary to lesions of the cauda equina. It has been found necessary by some surgeons to

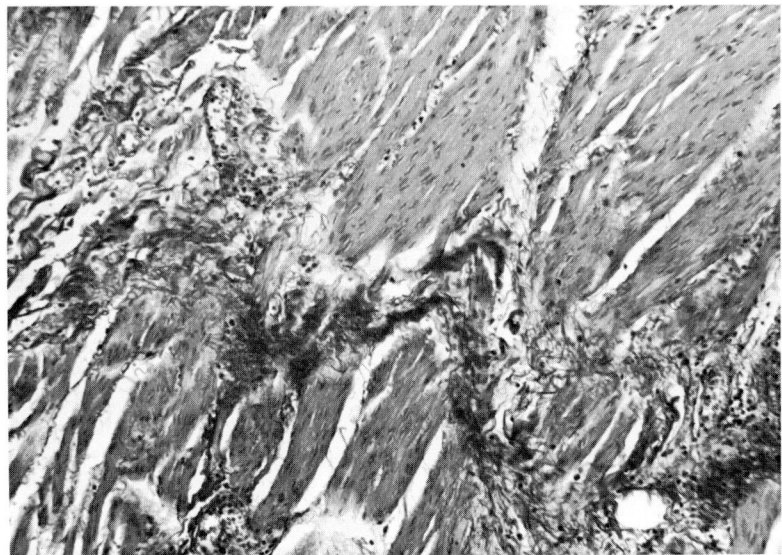

FIG. 47. Fibroelastic repair of sheared smooth-muscle bundles in the detrusor of a patient with interstitial cystitis. Note the spindling of smooth muscle fascicles adjacent to the area of scarring (center). Perimysial elastosis is absent. There is no evidence of elastosis within muscle fascicles or adjacent to individual muscle cells. Verhoeff-van Gieson stain. Original magnification X100.

revise the vesical neck, either transurethrally or by Y-V vesicourethroplasty, in association with operations designed to attack the primary obstructive process (Leadbetter and Leadbetter[304, 541]). It is evident from a study of the histotopographic anatomy that division of the ventral detrusor loop to convert the vesical neck into an anatomical funnel reduces the total resistance of the sphincteric urethra quite markedly.[437,185,544,191] It has become increasingly clear, however, that vesical-neck obstruction due to hypertrophy of the detrusor and trigonal loop mechanisms as a primary cause probably exists only in cases of neuromuscular dysfunction.

Hypertrophy of the bladder is a clinical anatomical and pathological term which has not been properly defined on an ultrastructural or molecular level. Light microscopy does little more than confirm its gross appearance.

The principal microscopic features in simple hypertrophy of the smooth-muscle bundle and fascicular structure are (1) some slight thickening of the intermuscular bundle collagen septa, (2) increase in the volume of muscle bundles due to increased volume of individual smooth-muscle cells, and (3) increase in random elastin fibers not associated with fibrosis or with perimysial or endomysial collagen (Fig. 48). Hypertrophy can exist side by side with markedly atrophic bundles in cases of partial neurogenic deficit (myelomeningocele). The content and distribution of elastin vary widely. In some cases of long-standing obstruction, *perimysial-bundle* elastin shows a marked increase. Interfascicular elastin may be increased without noticeable loss of smooth-muscle cell content.

Urethral Polyps

The term *congenital polyps of the prostatic urethra* was suggested by Downs[120] in his recent thorough review of the literature and the report of two additional cases, bringing the number of reported cases to 30 by February of 1970. The overall incidence is probably greater than this. In one series[345] four cases were identified in 600 voiding cystourethrograms, although Rudhe[447] found no polyps in his series of 2,000 voiding cystourethrograms. Downs suggests this term in that these polypoid lesions, occurring predominantly in infants and children, are of varying histological pattern.

These are not to be confused with the inflammatory polyps seen

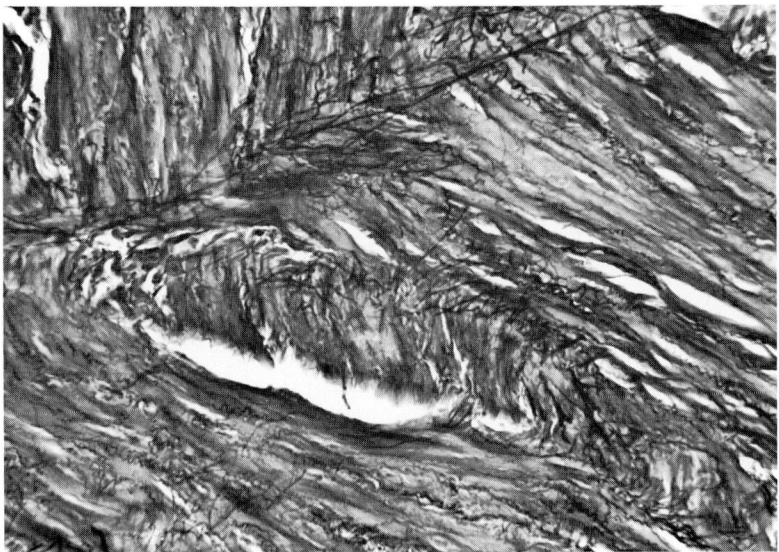

FIG. 48. Photomicrograph of bladder wall biopsy showing hypertrophy. Smooth-muscle cells are relatively large. There is a marked increase in rather randomly oriented elastic fibers (black) without accompanying increase in collagen. Verhoeff-van Gieson stain. Original magnification X250.

in both the female and male urethra and the structure of which is largely submucosal edema, epithelial metaplasia and infiltration with inflammatory cells; nor should they be confused with the aberrant prostatic epithelium noted by Nesbit in adult males.[378] Most frequently congenital polyps consist of a transitional-cell mucosal covering and vascularized fibrous connective-tissue core, and have been found to contain smooth muscle,[353,151] nerves and mucous glands,[478] as well as glandular cell nests. Occasionally squamous metaplasia of the epithelium is noted. The classical polyp arises above the verumontanum on the dorsal wall of the prostatic urethra. The body lies along the floor of the urethra and its tip protrudes toward the bladder neck (Fig. 49).

The mechanism of obstruction is due to its size and also to its impaction into the midsphincteric urethra during urination.[13] The reason for including it as a congenital lesion is that most cases have been reported in male infants and children under the age of 8 years, the youngest being 7 months. There is no comparable lesion reported in female infants and children.

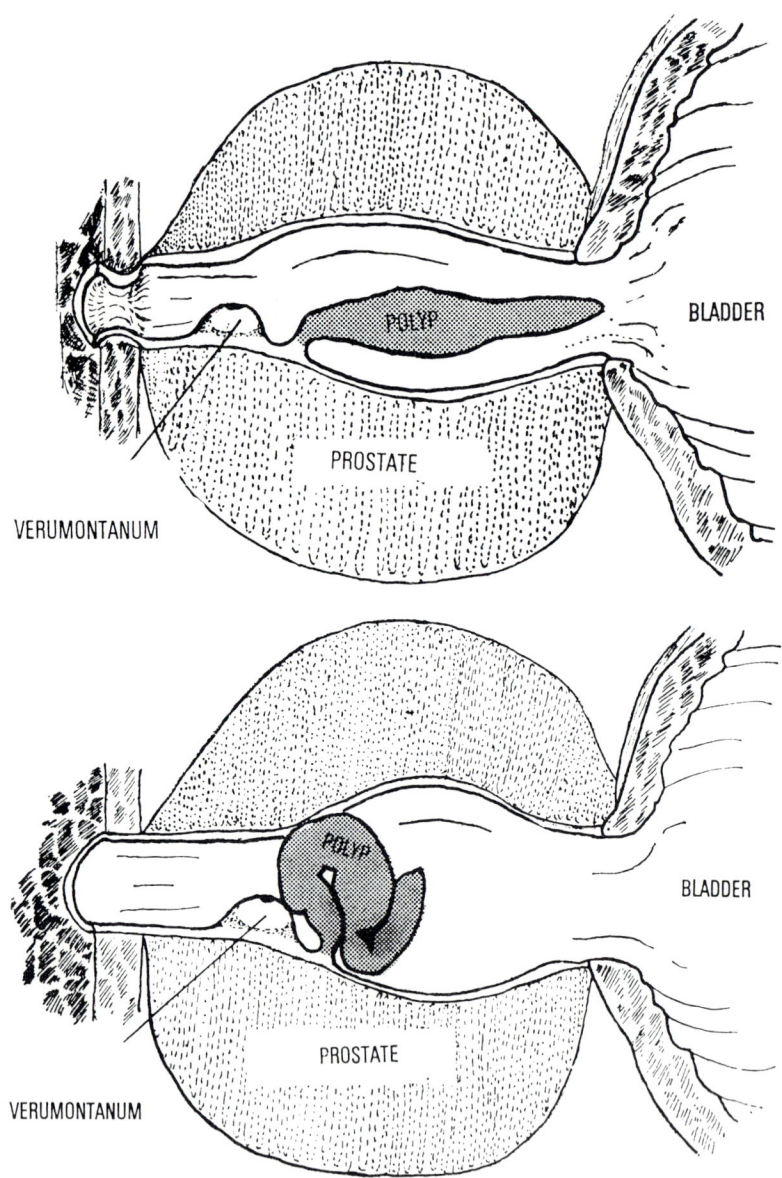

FIG. 49. Drawing to demonstrate the most frequent site of urethral polyp formation and the method by which it obstructs the sphincteric urethra. (Courtesy of Ralph A. Downs.)

The radiological appearance is characteristic; the rounded filling defect in the proximal sphincteric urethra buckling on itself during voiding is diagnostic. Congenital cysts of the vesical neck, ectopic ureteroceles or ectopic ureters opening in this position can cause some diagnostic confusion. However, careful urological study preoperatively usually clarifies the diagnosis and indicates the correct surgical approach.

Urethral Diverticulum

Anterior urethral valve is the term which has been largely applied to the distal ventral lip of a congenital urethral diverticulum of the pendulous urethra.[545,103,94,524] The most frequent site of this urethral obstruction is just proximal to the penoscrotal junction.[231] It should be remembered that, embryologically, the phallic portion of the urogenital sinus unites ventrally by infolding and fusion to form the bulbous urethra in a progressively distal manner toward the coronal sulcus.

Diverticula of the convex margin of the bulbous urethra may be confused with cystic dilatation of Cowper's ducts.[254,363] Cowper's duct cysts, which are often multiple, can be demonstrated by retrograde urethrography and are only rarely obstructive. Edling[128] makes a sharp distinction between diverticula in the posterior cavernous urethra and those in the pendulous urethra.

It has been proposed[262] that anterior urethral diverticula of this congenital nature are due to fusion failures, perhaps associated with incomplete development of the corpus spongiosum. An alternate proposal is that of Suter[481] and F. P. Johnson,[254] who feel that diverticula can arise from congenital cystic dilatations of the peri-urethral glands or from degenerated epidermal-cell nests. The valvular appearance most frequently noted at the distal end of the diverticulum is due, according to Williams and Retik,[545] to an upward displacement of the distal diverticular lip against the dorsal wall of the urethra, which then obstructs it. Narrow-necked diverticula are not ordinarily associated with this distal-lip type of obstructive valve formation, but do tend to become the site of infection and stone formation. Williams suggests that megalo-urethra and abortive urethral duplication may be variations in the embryogenesis of urethral diverticula and, as such, related to anterior valve formation. Anterior urethral valves and diverticula are relatively rare. Valvular obstruction due to posterior urethral valves occurs approximately ten times as frequently. In Williams' series of 17 cases, 8 patients were admitted to the hospital before the age of two years and 4 before the age of two weeks. Proximal damage to the urinary tract, including hypertrophied bladder, hydroureteronephrosis and renal failure, is less common in these lesions than with lesions in the region of the sphincteric urethra, and the results of surgical treatment are quite satisfactory.

Cysts

Cowper's-duct Cysts

Elbogen (1885) reported 15 cases of cysts of Cowper's ducts in a series of 645 autopsies.[132] Edling in 1953 reported 31 cases of cysts of the posterior urethra, 24 of which were located on the posterior wall in the region of Cowper's-duct orifices.[128] The cysts were smooth walled; some showed multiple cystic dilatations of the duct. The smallest cyst was 1 × 6 mm, the largest 30 × 60 mm. Numerous sporadic cases have been reported.[268,140,254,363,310,100,149] Anomalous absence of Cowper's glands has been mentioned (Cook and Shaw).

The most comprehensive review is that of Cook and Shaw.[100] The bulbo-urethral glands were originally described by Méry in 1684, but the first written description was by William Cowper in 1699.[101] Lebreton[310] in 1904 wrote a much-quoted monograph in which he described the development of the bulbo-urethral glands as side buds from the pelvic segment of the urogenital sinus visible in the 3- to 4-month fetus (50 to 112 mm). Johnson[254] described their presence in the 65-mm human fetus, and Arey[8] notes their first appearance in the 40-mm (10-week) fetus. Bloomfield and Fraser[26] identified Bartholin's-gland rudiments in one 28-mm embryo. In my embryological material the ducts and glands are quite apparent in the 55-mm embryo.

Necropsy specimens of Cowper's-duct cysts have not been commonly reported.

In the Anatomical Collection of Professor S. Gil Vernet, Series K, No. 4, there were 119 serial sections of the urethra, Cowper's-duct cysts, prostate, vesical neck and trigone made in the horizontal plane. Professor Gil Vernet was kind enough to allow me to review these sections and provided me with ten step sections, some of which are described and reproduced here (Figs. 50, 51, 52).

S. Gil Vernet reported that the specimen was brought to him from an autopsy in progress in the year 1940, with no clinical history and no upper urinary tract connected to the block of perineal tissue. The block of tissue included the rectum, a portion of the bladder, penis, scrotum and testes. The cephalad portion of the specimen terminated with the trigone. Two photographs of the gross specimen were available. They were difficult to interpret but showed a dilated segment of bladder, with a rather thin-walled appearance. The penis and testicles, and the pubic symphysis, which had been dissected, had the appearance of those belonging to a 6- or 7-year-old boy. Gross

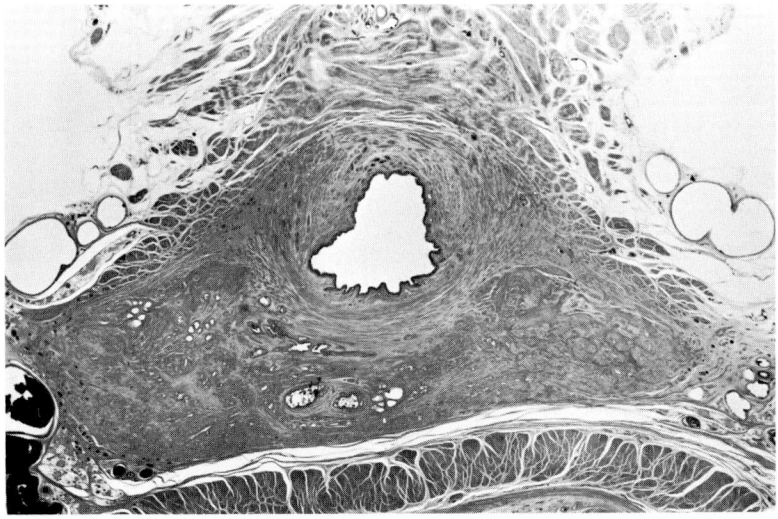

FIG. 50. Histotopographic appearance of dilated vesical neck in a 7-year-old boy as a result of bulbous urethral obstruction by Cowper's duct cysts. The cranial prostate can be seen beneath the trigonal loop fibers. Detrusor loop and transverse precervical arc bundles can be identified. There appears to be no hypertrophy of these bundles, but simply wide dilatation of the vesical neck. Hematoxylin-eosin-orange G (thick section 15 μ). Original magnification X10.

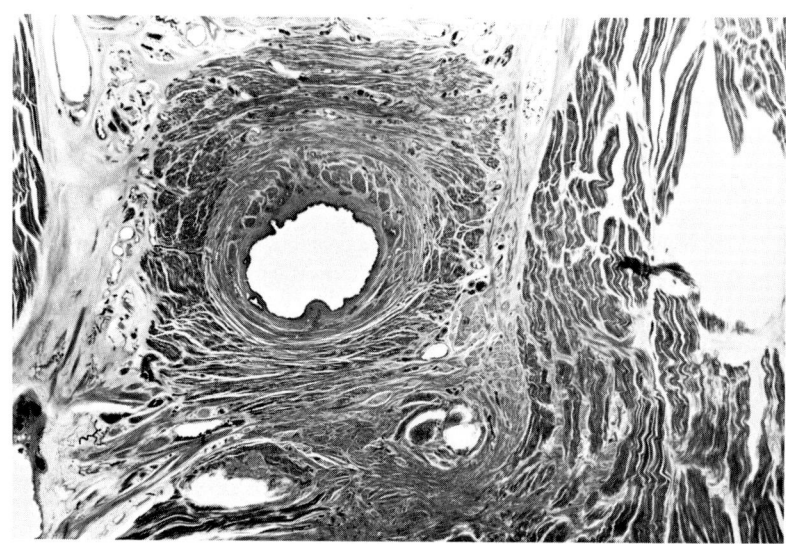

FIG. 51. Histotopographic appearance of membranous urethra in 7-year-old boy. Dilated lumen is secondary to distal obstruction by Cowper's duct cysts. Both Cowper's glands can be seen in this plane of section (lower center). Both are dilated and show structural loss and mucosal compression. Membranous urethral musculature is well defined. Intrinsic striated sphincter fibers more densely stained than smooth-muscle components. Hematoxylin-eosin-orange G stain. Original magnification X15.

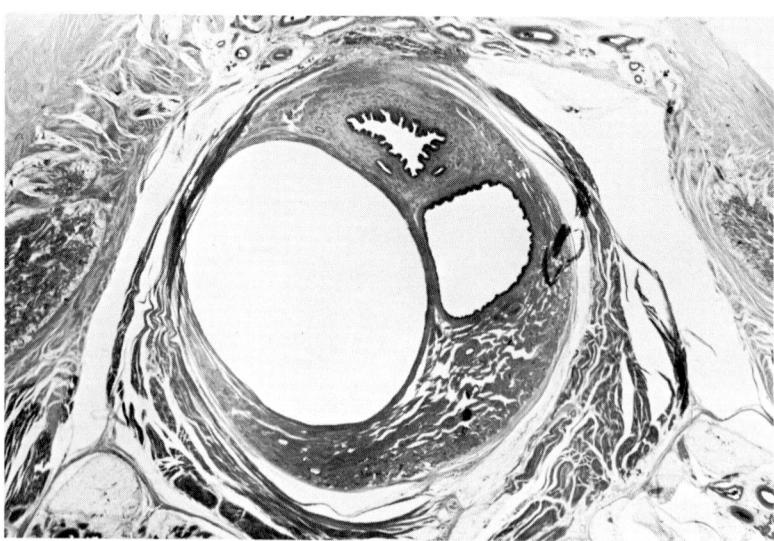

FIG. 52. Histotopographic section through bulbous urethra of 7-year-old boy to show massive cystic dilatation of Cowper's ducts within the corpora cavernosae. The distal portions of the ducts are in the same plane of section and lie immediately adjacent and below the compressed urethra (center top). Hematoxylin-eosin-orange G stain. Original magnification X5.

dissection of the specimen and embedding were carried out by Professor Gil Vernet. He described the section as being initially a puzzle. After trimming the specimen, he made a series of cautious, partial transverse incisions into the urethra. With one such incision made into the bulbous portion of the urethra, he was astounded to discover a jelly-like substance apparently occluding the urethra. When this was wiped from the surface, he noted what he thought to be a greatly dilated urethra. Subsequent sections through the prostate and vesical neck revealed no further abnormalities except for the dilated sphincteric urethra and vesical neck. The rectum showed no abnormalities, either grossly or upon serial section. There were no smooth-bundle muscular anomalies noted in the musculature of either the rectum or urethra. There were no apparent vascular anomalies. The distribution of nerves, histologically, within the pelvis was not abnormal. Sections were made of the entire trimmed block in a horizontal, slightly oblique, plane to include rectum, perineal musculature, prostate and urethra. Formalin-fixed sections were frozen and sectioned at thicknesses of approximately 15 to 20 μ. The sections were stained with hemotoxylin and eosin.

In reviewing the sections, passing from the base (interureteric ridge) of the trigone distally, one has the feeling that a single, more cephalad section would have included the ureteral orifices. Periureteral fiber bundles pass forward to become a portion of the trigonal musculature. The normal anatomical structure of the trigone, including trigonal loop, deep trigone, superficial trigonal muscle, is attenuated and does not appear to be reduced in substance, but merely distended (Fig. 50). There is marked dilation of the entire sphincteric urethra. A section through the membranous urethra includes the obstructed and dilated Cowper's glands (Fig. 51).

There were actually cysts of *both* Cowper's ducts. The larger one was 6 × 8 mm in diameter, the smaller one approximately 1 mm. The larger cyst almost completely replaced the corpora cavernosa at this point (Fig. 52). Measurements of the diameter of Buck's fascia in two planes is 14 mm in width and 13 mm in the ventrodorsal axis. The dorsally situated urethra is displaced and compressed by surrounding tissue.

Müllerian-duct Cysts

Müllerian-duct cysts as a cause of infravesical obstruction are relatively uncommon. Neustein and Schutte in 1968[380] collected 55 cases from the literature. They credit Englisch in 1873[139] with the first report of müllerian-duct cyst in a stillborn. In all, Englisch reported 5 cases in 70 newborn males.

Müllerian-duct cysts can become quite large without producing major obstruction, because they are analogous to the müllerian portion of the vagina, and the cystic enlargement is therefore always posterior to the proximal sphincteric urethra. These cysts usually appear as cystic masses beneath the trigone. Symptoms of secondary infection, rather than primarily those of obstruction, ordinarily call these to the attention of the physician. F. S. Howard in 1948[233] demonstrated utricular enlargement in 10 of 14 cases of hypospadias. These included two cases in which a vagina and uterus were found. Young and Cash in 1921[564] reported a müllerian-duct cyst in a male pseudohermaphrodite. As Howard suggests, persistence of an enlarged utricle or utricular-cyst formation indicates some degree of feminization of the embryo, and in the more dramatic cases this shades gradually into the realm of the intersexes. The cysts may contain calculi, even in children.[469] The fact that müllerian-duct cysts are not usually obstructing in the infant and child is borne out by the fact that exceedingly large cysts have been reported, ordinarily in adult males or in males of the prostatic-hypertrophy age group, particularly by Moore and Howe[354] and Neustein and Schutte.[380] This is not actually one of the "obscure" vesical-neck obstructions in childhood, and the diagnosis can frequently be better made by rectal examination than by voiding cystourethrography or cystoscopy. The diagnosis should be considered, however, in male children with urinary infection and obstructive symptoms.[127,409] One of the most interesting embryological variations of a müllerian-duct cyst is the case reported by Ceccarelli and Beach[82] in which a unilateral persistent müllerian duct was found attached to the mesonephros of a young adult male, in which all three embryological renal generations were present.

Megacystis

Obstruction to the outflow of urine from the bladder in children can be mimicked by conditions in which actual mechanical obstruction is absent but in which a functional imbalance of the detrusor and sphincteric mechanism is present. Classically, this occurs in some cases of myelomeningocele with myelodysplasia in which there is a deficit in the autonomic or somatic nerve supply to the bladder musculature and sphincteric urethra. "Megacystis" is not quite an honorable diagnosis (DeLuca, et al.,[111] Harrow[216]); it has, however, been frequently reported.[282, 130, 315, 191, 569] Idiopathic dilatation of other visceral organs invested by smooth muscle is not uncommon. O'Wilensky,[387] in an excellent review, discussed the "mega" syndromes. Megaduodenum, megagastrium, megacolon and megaesophagus are well recognized. Achalasia of the esophagus can even be supported with electron-microscopic evidence of disordered "grapple plaques"—possibly the sites of smooth-muscle myosin—on the inner surfaces of the plasma membranes of the muscle cells (Harman, O'Hegarty and Byrnes[213]). A perhaps similar imbalance is recognized in the syndrome of "megacystis," in which there is evident hypotonia of the detrusor musculature (Fig. 53). A microscopic lesion can be described in some of the children exhibiting these large, thin-walled bladders with reduced expulsive force which appears to be a lesion of smooth muscle.

Megacystis is a clincial syndrome clearly defined by D. Innes-Williams[537] in 1954, of which the primary feature is a large-capacity bladder exhibiting hypotonia and rigidity of the detrusor musculature and in which there is no evidence of neurological involvement of the somatic musculature. The bladder shadow, on cystography, reaches the fifth lumbar vertebra or above it twice as frequently as normal (Jones and Headstream[257]). The trigone is ordinarily widened[390] and ureteral reflux is quite uniformly present.[538, 539, 474]

Cystometrograms frequently demonstate moderate hypotonia with a sudden rise in intravesical pressure at ultimate capacity, upon which Paquin, Marshall and McGovern[390] commented ". . . as if the elasticity in the bladder wall were somewhat impaired."

As in most clinical syndromes, all of these signs may not be present in impressive degree in an individual case. Residual urine can be surprisingly absent or, if present, may be small in amount.

Negative diagnostic signs, that is, the *absent* findings, are probably of as much importance as positive ones. These include: (1) absence of demonstrable neurological lesions involving the somatic lumbo-sacral outflow of the spinal cord, (2) absence of demonstrable infravesical obstruction on cinecystourethrography or at cystoscopy, (3)

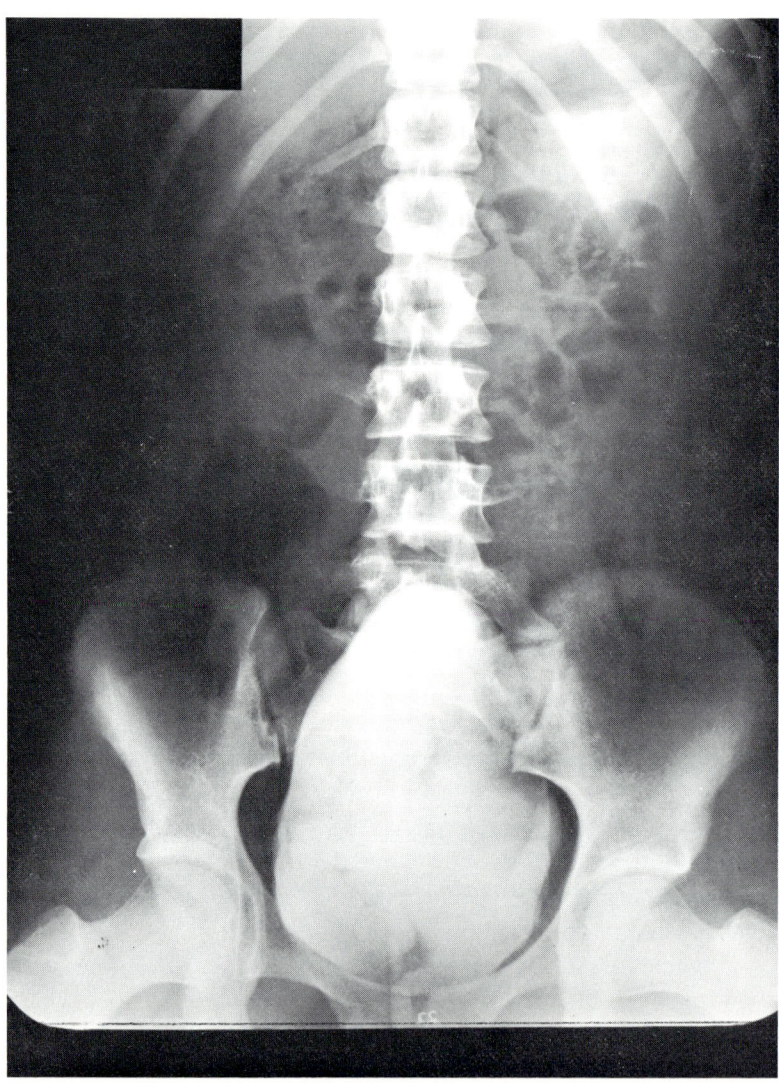

FIG. 53. Case 1 (C.H.), 17-year-old girl. Cystogram showing greatly enlarged hypotonic bladder and reflux into left ureteral stump. No reflux to right kidney following ureterovesical junction reconstruction. Note smooth bladder wall.

absence of heavy trabeculation of the bladder wall and the confirmation of extremely thin musculature of the detrusor at operation, (4) essentially normal intravesical pressures on voiding cystometrography, and (5) the observation that the vesical neck appears slightly rigid during early filling at cystoscopy, with no measureable stenosis, and then suddenly springs open to a relatively normal size at what may be a critical level of detrusor elasticity.

Studies of the underlying lesion in megacystis have been few. Swenson, et al.[484] in 1952 and Swenson and Fisher[483] in 1955 proposed an analogy of megacystis and megaureter to Hirschsprung's disease of the colon, and speculated upon a selective derangement of the pelvic parasympathetic nerves to account for the association of the two conditions in some cases. The histological evidence of decreased or absent ganglia and nerves within the detrusor muscle has not been thoroughly convincing and, in several cases of classical megacystis, Leibowitz and Bodian[314] found no diminution in the number of ganglion cells surrounding the bladder. Paquin, Marshall and McGovern[390] postulate a congenital anomaly producing a disproportion of the vesical base ("megatrigone") associated with thin detrusor musculature. This suggests the concept of a general *"dysgenesis"* of smooth muscle, which is a reasonable postulate. Scher[451] has reported selective *absence* of the superficial trigonal muscle. Harrow, Sloane and Wittus[215] have suspected some type of *muscular dysplasia* in congenital dilatation of the female urethra. Absent abdominal musculature in association with urinary tract abnormalities, including hypotonia of the detrusor, has been frequently reported,[384,320,385] and associated dysplasia of the detrusor musculature can be demonstrated in some of these cases. Henley and Hyman[222] propose, alternately, a defect in the pelvic autonomic nervous system as an underlying cause. Nunn and Stephens[384] suggest that the etiology of the "triad syndrome" is related to mesenchymal defects of the somatopleure. Stephens and Lenaghan have also postulated a dysplastic mesenchymal defect in the development of the juxtavesical longitudinal smooth muscle of the ureter to account for ureteral reflux.[474]

In the search for a biochemical etiology of megacystis, Rohner, et al.[438] have demonstrated an increase in the glycogen content of the smooth muscle of the denervated dog bladder and speculated that this might represent an influence upon the smooth-muscle phosphorylase enzyme system to produce a situation comparable to McArdle's disease in skeletal muscle, in which absent phosphorylase produces a classical myopathy.

Theoretically, intrauterine overdistension of the bladder with prenatal rupture of the muscle bundles, and their subsequent repair, might be considered in the production of these large, thin-walled, hypotonic bladders, and it is conceivable that prenatal infravesical obstruction of a transient nature could have been the underlying cause. Functional retention in older children may further confuse the diagnosis. It might also be considered that the bladder tone in cases of megacystis may have been altered by an autoimmune or inflammatory process. McDonald, et al.[367] reported 45 cases of interstitial cystitis in children, predominantly female, who exhibited *contracted* bladders. These authors made no mention of muscle or fibroelastic lesions in their material.

The possibility that megacystis may represent a primary disease of smooth muscle has not been seriously considered; perhaps it should be.

Involvement of smooth-muscle in association with skeletal-muscle myopathies is being reported with increasing frequency. Pruzanski and Huvos[421,249] have demonstrated focal and patchy necrosis with hypereosinophilia of smooth-muscle myofibers in the esophagus, stomach, colon and urinary bladder in association with progressive muscular dystrophy; they have also described degenerative lesions of the bladder musculature in amyotonic dystrophy and myasthenia gravis.[248]

Degenerative disease of smooth muscle was also reported in the bowel and esophagus in extensive progressive muscular dystrophy by Bevans.[22] Bunting[63] in 1908 noted associated lesions in the smooth muscle of the stomach in which numerous fascicles showed numerical atrophy of fibers and invasion by connective tissue. Some remaining fibers were vacuolated and degenerated in appearance, while others appeared hypertrophied. In the cases reported by Bevans, examination of smooth muscle of the prostate, bladder and epididymis showed no abnormalities. In one case, examination of the striated muscle of the urinary sphincter showed degenerative changes similar to dystrophic lesions in the striated muscle. Changes in cardiac muscle have been reported in association with muscular dystrophy,[57] and isolated cardiomyopathy has been reported in pregnancy.[98]

The proportions of viable, contractile smooth-muscle cells to collagen and elastin within the detrusor are of the utmost importance in maintaining the integrity of the detrusor-sphincteric function. This is probably a most significant functional factor in megacystis. Cussen[106] has made quantitative microscopic measurements of the *ureteral* smooth muscle in the normal human ureter during the first twelve years of life. Stein and Weinberg[471] applied similar semiquanitative measurements to the smooth-muscle coats of the ureter by using a filar micrometer eyepiece, and then microscopically measured and averaged the thickness of the muscle coats compared with the thickness of the ureteral wall. They estimated the amount of collagen and elastin present in a series of infant, adult, and animal ureters and found the amount of muscle in the normal adult ureteral wall to be approximately 50 percent of the total tissue components, and slightly less at birth. They surmised that the amount of muscle in the ureter decreased in acute obstruction and increased with chronic obstruction, suggesting hypertrophy. They found no decrease in the amount of smooth muscle in the *megaureters* studied.

Bradley, Chou, Markland and Swaiman[45] were able accurately to estimate the amount of fibrosis in the bladder by means of bio-assay of collagenous protein as a percentage of total bladder-wall protein. Histological assay of the fibrous-tissue formation was not as reliable an indicator of bladder-wall sclerosis as was the biochemical method in their experimental series.

In the course of the histological studies upon which this monograph is based, four cases of megacystis were encountered and intensively studied by light microscopy. Biochemical assay techniques were unfortunately unavailable. A common histological change was noted in each of these cases which was unlike mural changes due to other pathological processes affecting the bladder musculature; although resembling the myopathies closely, it had certain features which may be singular to the musculature of the urinary bladder.

Full-thickness biopsy specimens from the dome and vesical neck or lower third of the bladder wall were obtained from the patients during the course of reconstructive surgery (ages 3, $4\frac{1}{2}$, 5 and 17 years), each of whom exhibited this type of nonobstructive, hypotonic, smooth-wall bladder dysfunction. Specimens were prepared for microscopic examination and stained with Verhoeff-van Gieson, Luxol fast-blue-PAS, Luxol fast-blue-Holmes' silver nitrate, Bielschowsky's silver, Masson's trichrome, hematoxylin-eosin-PAS and phosphotungstic acid-hematoxylin (PTAH).

Similar staining techniques and examinations were carried out from recut blocks of biopsies in 18 infants, children and adults (Table 4). Six were clinically normal. Pathological material examined included: neurogenic bladder (2), mechanical obstruction (6), hypertrophy (2), interstial cystitis (1), smooth-muscle dysplasia (triad syndrome) (1).

TABLE 4. *Vesical Biopsies—Control Series*

	Patient	Age and Sex	Diagnosis
1.	Baby—Y15-66 (PMC)	8-mo. Fetus—F	Normal
2.	Baby—I-B5-HZ (U.I.)	Stillborn—M	Obstruction—Vesical Neck
3.	Baby—I-U.K. BH-9 (U.I.)	Stillborn—M	Obstruction—"Valves"
4.	Baby—Y-18-67 (PMC)	Stillborn—F	Normal
5.	Baby—Y-17-67 (PMC)	Stillborn—M	Normal
6.	A.M.—A268-67 (BGH)	17 days—M	Triad Syndrome
7.	T.P.—A66-110 (PMC)	4 wks.—M	Normal
8.	B-H-1—(U.I.)	2 yrs.—M	Normal
9.	G.N.—A64-98 (PMC)	3 yrs.—M	Normal
10.	F.N.—S-62-1569 (PMC)	5 yrs.—M	Myelomeningocele (Lower Motor Neuron)
11.	J.C.—P218878 (PMC)	5 yrs.—F	Hypertrophy—Cystitis
12.	S.B.—S-1605-B (PMC)	5½ yrs.—F	Obstruction—Vesical Neck
13.	M.G.—S-65-1423 (PMC)	8 yrs.—M	Hypertrophy (Postencephalitis ?)
14.	T.B.—S-66-2729 (PMC)	40 yrs.—M	Neurogenic Bladder (Upper Motor Neuron)
15.	G.P.—S-1928-A (PMC)	42 yrs.—M	Obstruction—Vesical Neck
16.	G.M.—S-61-1771 (PMC)	44 yrs.—F	Interstitial Cystitis
17.	I.B.—N.G.4-8755 (NGH)	58 yrs.—F	Obstruction—Diverticula
18.	Y-2-1—A64-212 (PMC)	80 yrs.—F	Fibrosis—Atrophy

Photomicrographs and drawings were made of significant sections, and detailed descriptions and comparisons were carried out. Further careful family histories were taken in cases showing muscular lesions, with particular regard to genetic aspects of skeletal-muscle disease. Serum levels of aldolase, creatine phosphokinase and LDH isoenzymes were obtained in each of the megacystis patients and in the entire family of one patient. All serum enzyme studies were within normal limits.

HISTOLOGICAL LESION

The histological lesion in these cases consisted of a segmental replacement of portions of smooth-muscle fascicles throughout the detrusor by a floccular, eosinophilic ground substance associated with a substantial, probably secondary[205,265] elastosis (Figs. 54*A*, *B*, *C* and *D*). Grossly, the bladders showed a smooth mucosa with minimal trabeculation. The average bladder-wall thickness was less than 0.75 cm. The mucosa was intact throughout and no ulcerations or localized thickenings were noted. In one case there was a disparity in the

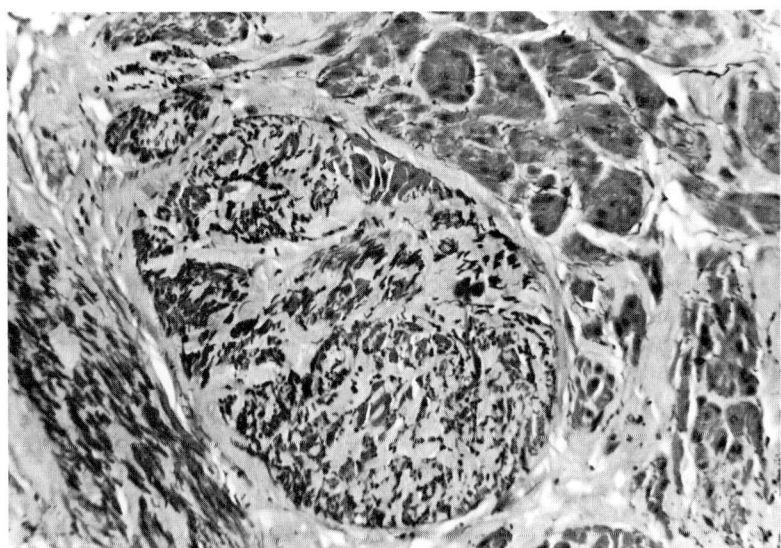

FIG. 54. *A*, Smooth-muscle lesion in megacystis. Muscle bundle (center) shows marked random segmental fascicular degeneration with striking elastic fiber replacement. Intermuscular bundle septa thickened and glassy. There are several remaining smooth-muscle cells near the upper margin. Relatively normal bundle upper right. Note absence of leukocytes. Verhoeff-van Gieson stain. Original magnification X250.

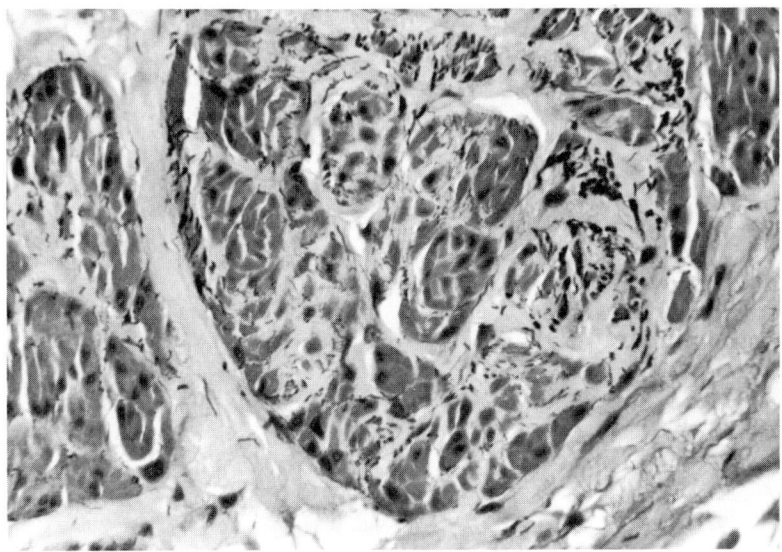

B, Varying degrees of fascicular degeneration within a single smooth-muscle bundle. Fascicles at left and center show loss of cellular structure and floccular hyaline replacement. Transversely sectioned elastic fibers are prominent in fascicles at right. Note thickened septa (endomysium) between fascicles. Verhoeff-van Gieson stain. Original magnification X400.

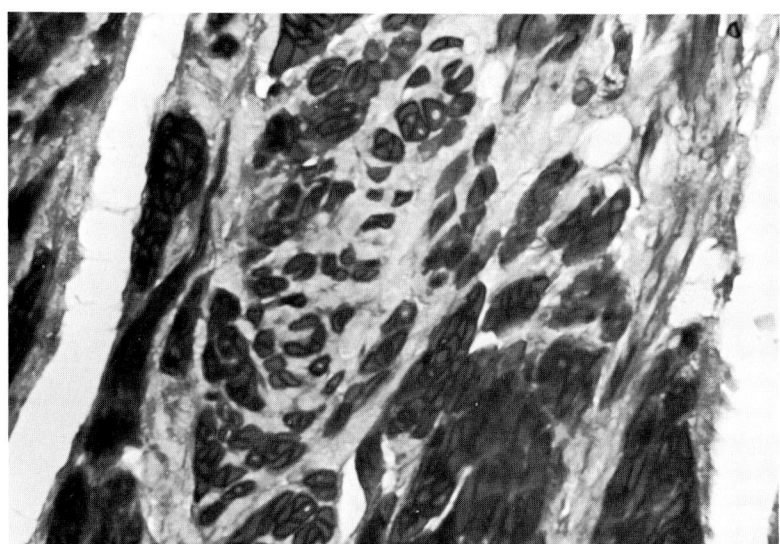

FIG. 54. *C*, Smooth-muscle fascicle with areas of smooth-muscle cell degeneration. Luxol fast-blue-PAS stain. Original magnification X400.

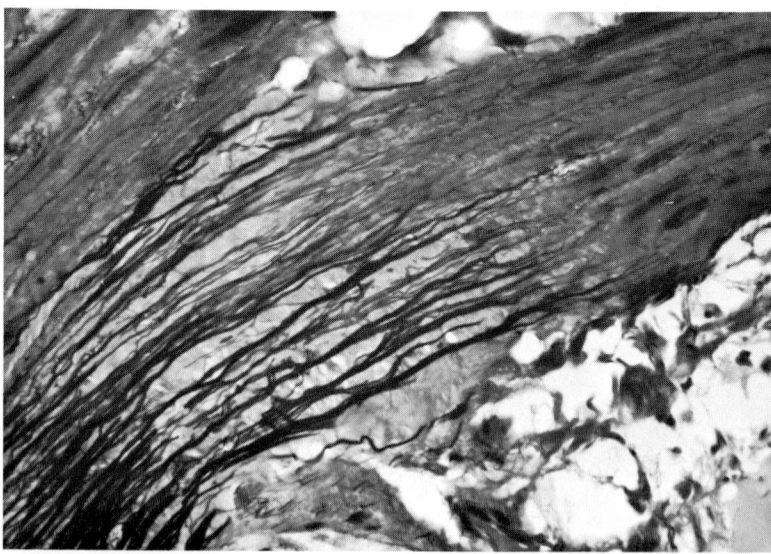

D, "Junctional zone" between normal smooth-muscle and area of floccular hyaline replacement. Here smooth-muscle cells lose their structural characteristics and staining properties, become swollen and vacuolar. Elastic fibers interdigitate in parallel with the bordering muscle cells. Verhoeff-van Gieson stain. Original magnification X400.

thickness of the dome of the bladder and the base. The base showed slight trabeculation and measured almost 1.0 cm in thickness, while the dome was perfectly smooth and half the thickness of the base. Interestingly enough, the "replaced" muscle, histologically, was markedly less in the dome than in the bladder base.

In areas of the most severe involvement, muscle bundles were isolated from one another by a greatly increased intramuscular bundle deposition of edematous, eosinophilic material mingled with collagen fibers. These, the former intermuscular bundle septae (perimysium), showed random elastic fibers, dilated lymphatics, areas of closely grouped fat cells, but no infiltration of leukocytes and only rare macrophages. Vesical biopsies from other sites showed less intermuscular-bundle edema and fibrosis, but the random intrafascicular smooth-muscle lesions and replacement were frequently as pronounced within an individual bundle as in the most edematous portions.

Contiguous fascicles were not involved at precisely the same sites, or to the same degree, within a muscle bundle. The lesion was neither central nor peripheral within a muscle bundle, but seemed to occur at random. The lesion was present in both the base and vertex of the bladder. The lesion, significantly, was not present in the juxta-vesical ureteral smooth muscle in one case, in which marked changes were present in the bladder. Normal nerve bundles and adventitial ganglia could be identified, not only in relatively uninvolved portions of the muscle but also in areas of severe degeneration, where hyaline material, deposition fibrosis, and fatty replacement had taken place (Fig. 55). There were no changes in the intima, media or external elastic layers of arteries. No perivascular inflammatory infiltrate could be identified. Crystal violet and the Benhold's Congo-red stain for amyloid were negative.

The mucosa and tunica propria were intact but edematous, and in one case were infiltrated with leukocytes. There was a prominent increase in PAS-positive granular material in the *junctional zones*, apparently related to the disintegrated cytolemma of individual smooth-muscle cells. An increase in the perinuclear clear space with concomitant decrease in cytoplasmic myofibrils was associated with darkly stained and clumped smooth-muscle nuclei.

A striking feature of the lesions within the bladder was the marked associated elastosis. This is probably not specific for these lesions as it was seen in the perimysial and endomysial connective tissue in cases

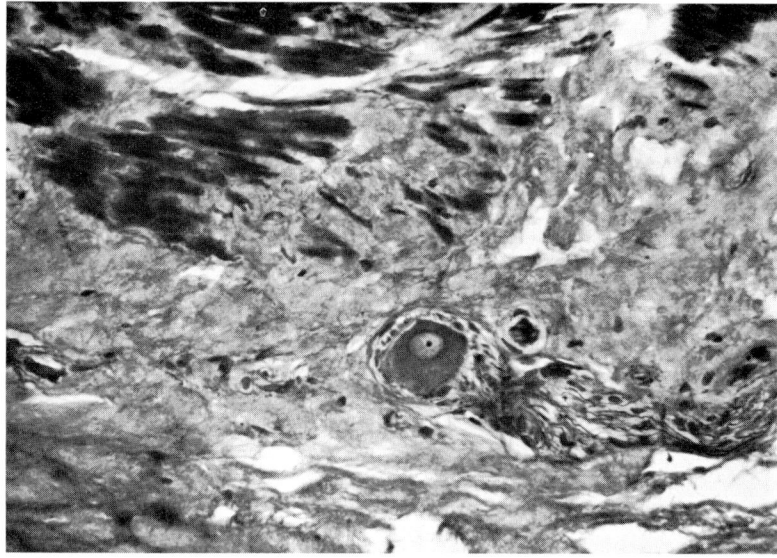

FIG. 55. Intact ganglion cell and nerve (center right) in area of extensive degeneration. Smooth-muscle cells at upper left show fragmentation, structural loss and hyaline replacement. Luxol fast-blue-Holmes' silver nitrate stain. Original magnification X400.

of hypertrophy and long-standing obstruction, as well as in the neurogenic bladder, and is part of random fibroelastic replacement tissue in ruptured muscle bundles noted in interstitial cystitis.

Longitudinal sections of the smooth-muscle cells, when examined at higher powers, showed that the areas of degeneration form junctional regions with normal smooth-muscle cells at both ends. These junctional regions were of interest, for here the sarcoplasm of individual smooth-muscle cells loses its fibrillary appearance and staining characteristics and becomes glassy, swollen and floccular. Coarse, discrete, blunt-ended elastic fibers bridging the lesion pass between the smooth-muscle cells bordering the lesion for 20 to 30 μ on either side of the area of destruction. Nuclei become darkened and crowded together within the fascicle on PTAH stain. Within the lesion itself there are no leukocytes, no smooth-muscle nuclei, and no argyrophillic structures to suggest nerve endings or reticular fibers. There were only occasional macrophages. Definite myoblasts have not been identified. The replacement elastic fibers are all arranged longitudinally with relation to the involved smooth-muscle cells and appear to conform to the lines of force originally established by the fascicle.

Histologically, the lesion identified at both the dome and in the lower third of the urinary bladder in these four children was identical. Specifically, it did not resemble patterns of hypertrophy, obstruction, lower or upper motor-neuron deficit, interstitial cystitis or dysplasia. Blood vessels, ganglia and nerve bundles could be identified, even in the areas of extensive degeneration. There seemed to be neither an increase or decrease in the number of adventitial or perimysial ganglion cells, as compared with the normal.

Features of this lesion of smooth muscle suggest myopathy: cloudy swelling of the cells and the loss of myofibrillar structure, interstitial edema, lymphatic prominence and presence of macrophages. Vacuolization of the smooth-muscle cells is present and the vacuolated cells frequently show an associated pyknosis and hyperchromatism of the nucleus.

The segmental and random nature of this smooth-muscle lesion with no evidence of inflammatory response and a relatively non-progressive clinical course suggests that the lesion is of established standing—perhaps prenatal. The presence of fascicles in various stages of architectural decay, on the other hand, is evidence against a primary dysplasia due to mesenchymal failure, and speaks for an active, if indolent, process of destruction and repair. Perhaps extraordinary stretching of a fascicle destroys or ruptures individual cells. Local ischemia, due to vesical distention, could account for this finding. The nature of the lesion seems to require some destructive event to account for this pattern of disintegration of segments of the preformed smooth-muscle fascicles.

The clinicopathological correlation is evident. Increased rigidity produced by the replacement of smooth-muscle cells with hyaline material and elastic fibers interposed in direct sequence within the smooth-muscle fascicles must, certainly, severely limit the wide, normal excursions of the contractility and distensibility of the smooth-muscle fascicles.

Vesical Dysplasia

The Triad ("Prune Belly") Syndrome (Eagle-Barrett)

William Osler[386] in 1901 reported a case of congenital absence of the abdominal muscles with a distended and hypertrophied urinary bladder, although the first description of this abnormality is attributed to Frölich[162] in 1839. Parker[393] in 1895 made the association among absent abdominal-wall musculature, undescended testicles and the urinary tract abnormalities. There have been excellent clinical reports and reviews of collected cases by Williams and Burkholder,[543] Lattimer,[303] Eagle-Barrett[123] and Silverman and Huang.[459]

The syndrome, by definition limited to males, carries a high infant mortality. Twenty percent of the 120 cases collected by Williams and Burkholder were stillborn or died within one month; 50 percent died within two years.

This bizarre association of anomalies may be accompanied by other systemic defects, most frequently skeletal, including pectus excavatum, congenital dislocation of the hip and talipes equinus. The gastrointestinal tract may be involved (Bruton[52]) and, rarely, the central nervous system (Lichtenstein[320]). A somewhat similar set of anomalies may exist in girls.[303,152,344,227] In girls, absent abdominal musculature often appears to be partial, the urinary tract abnormalities are not as severe, and the associated anomalies of other organ systems are much more striking (Williams and Burkholder[543]).

This association (of absent abdominal-wall musculature, undescended testicles and urinary tract abnormalities) is most often accompanied by a specific defect in the bladder. Bladders in these children are found to be thickened, though not trabeculated. Functionally they are lethargic, showing increased capacities and (inconstantly) residual urine. The vesical neck is apt to be lax and widely open at rest, allowing the proximal sphincteric urethra to be filled with urine. Abnormalities of the upper tract are not necessarily related to the hypotonia of the bladder. Williams,[537,538,539] Mogg[353] and Powell[412] have noted a widened trigone, persistent attachment of the urachus to the umbilicus, and occasionally a persistent umbilical urinary fistula.

Henley and Hyman[222] have suggested that this defect is due, as in megacystis, to a deficiency of the vesical ganglia. Secondary atrophy of the abdominal-wall musculature due to fetal overdistention of the bladder has again been, rather grandly, proposed as a cause. A third possibility postulated is primary urethral obstruction in fetal life.[192] Cystoscopic investigation of these children has rarely revealed well-documented evidence of any of the usual congenital obstructive lesions.[38,302]

Dysplasia of detrusor smooth muscle as an accompaniment to the dysplasia of the striated musculature of the abdominal wall has been suggested as an explanation for this condition.[472,475,470,546] The concept of a common mesenchymal failure, of undetermined fetal origin, is intriguing. Purely entodermal and ectodermal structures, i.e., the rectosigmoid, integument and genital tubercle, appear to be spared involvement in this symptom complex. The organs involved—kidney, bladder, ureter and testis (or possibly the gubernaculum testis)—all have as a common origin mesodermal elements of the dorsolateral body wall.

Ikeda and Stoesser[252] at autopsy reported dense fibrosis at the bladder wall. The histological studies of the bladder by Burkholder and Harper[64] in two cases have shown areas of focal fibrosis associated with reduction in amount of muscle. Specimens of bladder wall from each of these cases, which these authors kindly furnished for my examination, showed a similar and somewhat characteristic mural fibrosis with a loss of the normal perimysial-endomysial architecture and relationships of the muscle bundles associated with diffuse areas of fibrosis. This fibrosis was not associated with the marked elastosis seen in children's bladders with either long-standing obstructions or those resulting from neurogenic dysfunction. Many of the muscle fascicles contained only 8 or 10 smooth-muscle cells and were surrounded by islands of dense, well-formed collagen (Fig. 56*A, B*). The muscle cells themselves appeared to be intact. There was no evidence of *intrafascicular* degeneration. Nerves and one large ganglion containing five large ganglion cells were visible in the adventitia (Fig. 57). Fibrosis appeared to be more severe in the adventitial layers than in the deeper layers of the musculature. Many of the smooth muscle fascicles and the larger aggregates—comparable to the smooth-muscle bundles—showed a definite decrease in the number of muscle cells.

Sphincteric Hypotonia

There have been isolated, and well-documented, reports of what appears to be an *hypotonic functional obstruction* of the sphincteric urethra and detrusor in males with normal abdominal muscles and descended testes.[215,412] This has been described as *"wide-neck bladder obstruction."* Clinically, it is manifested by a widely opened vesical neck with a dilated sphincteric urethra, tapering gently to an apparently normal bulbomembranous urethra within the triangular ligament.

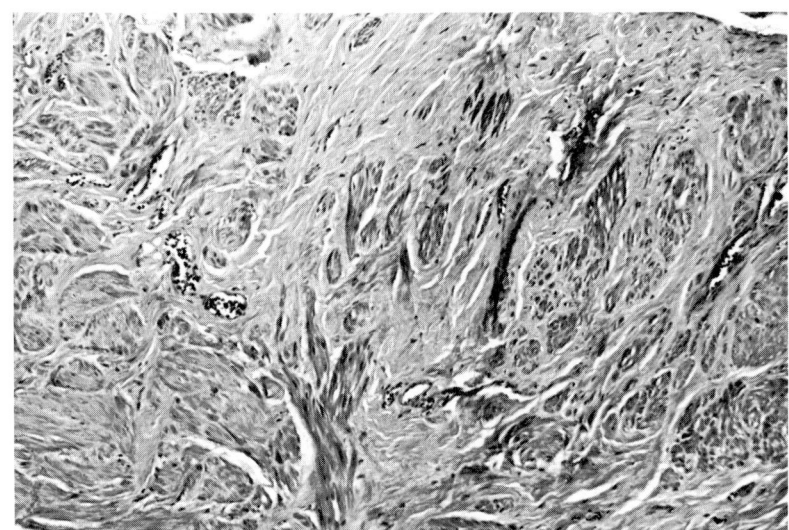

FIG. 56. (T.S.), Brooke General Hospital S-68-0776. Photomicrographs of detrusor muscle in a case of "triad syndrome." The smooth muscle of the bladder wall shows dysplasia. Marked disorganization of the normal architecture, a scarcity of smooth-muscle cells and dense collagen replacement (*A*). Elastosis is not a feature of this lesion (*B*). Verhoeff-van Gieson stain. Original magnifications X100 and X250. (Courtesy R. C. Harper and G. V. Burkholder.)

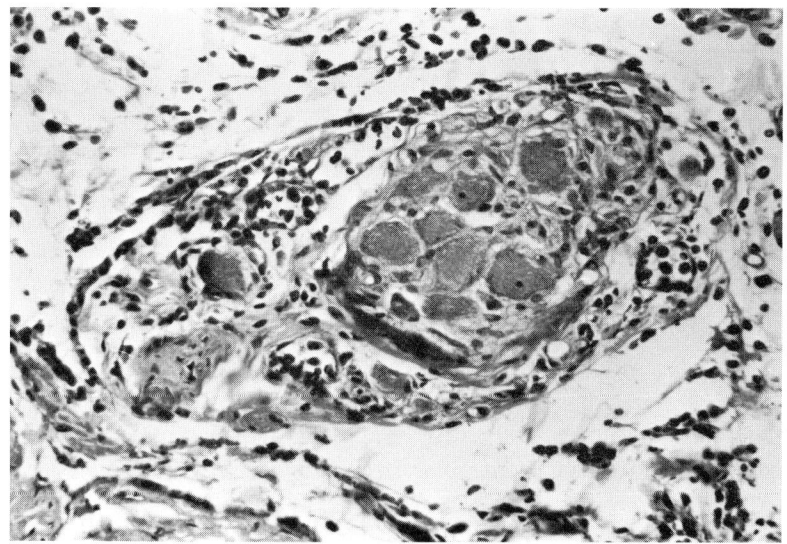

FIG. 57. (T.S.), Brooke General Hospital S-68-0776. Photomicrograph of adventitial ganglion from wall of dysplastic bladder in "triad syndrome." Structural details are not abnormal. The black, round cells are erythrocytes. Masson trichrome stain. Original magnification X250. (Courtesy of R. C. Harper and G. V. Burkholder.)

No primary obstructive lesion has been found.[546,492] The clinical features of this condition are akin to both megacystis and the hypotonic bladder seen in the "prune-belly" syndrome. The oldest child in Williams' series was six years, the youngest one week. The kidneys were anomalous in all cases. Ureters were dilated and reflux was universally present. Bladders were of large capacity and smooth walled, though at operation the muscle walls were of normal thickness. The bladders emptied slowly and residual urine was not a prominent feature. Stress incontinence and enuresis were the usual complaints. Voiding cystourethrograms showed the posterior urethra to be widely dilated, as was the vesical neck. Biopsy specimens in Williams' series failed to reveal fibroelastosis, nor in his cases were there obvious somatic neurological lesions.

It has been again suggested that this abnormality has a neurogenic basis.[150,72] In two of Williams' cases, wrinkling of the abdominal-wall skin was noted, suggesting some relation to the triad syndrome.[546] As an hypothesis, as King suggests,[269] it might be reasonable to suppose that this condition represents one of the *degrees* of mesenchymal dysplasia. It closely resembles the other idiopathic hypotonias affecting the detrusor musculature. The common histological features in all of these conditions are (1) marked fibrosis without elastosis, (2) the absence of normal amounts of smooth muscle and (3) architectural disarray of the smooth-muscle bundle structure.

Neurogenic Bladder

Within the context of this study, a detailed investigation of all of the facets of the neurogenic bladder in childhood could not be undertaken. Excellent and compendious reviews of this subject have been made available by Boyarsky,[39] Williams,[539] Bors,[37] Comar,[96] Nesbit and Lapides,[374] Prather[414] and Eckstein.[125] Current investigations of specific neuromuscular, contractile and transmission systems within the detrusor are being widely pursued.[45,46,47,328,454,200,341]

The principal reason for inclusion of a discussion of the neurogenic bladder here is to establish its relation to the other mechanical and functional lower urinary tract obstructive lesions producing similar clinical findings. Children with myelomeningocele or myelodysplasia, with lower motor-neuron lesions of unpredictable extent affecting the bladder, represent the great bulk of cases of neurogenic bladder. Bladder function in these children with undeterminable lesions of the cauda equina or sacral spinal cord is equally variant. Morphological changes in the bladder reflect the protean nature of the neurological lesion, so that it is difficult to anticipate in advance whether the bladder will show heavy trabeculation with diverticulum formation, secondary hypertrophy and large amounts of residual urine with upper tract damage, or whether it may be small and contracted with total urinary incontinence due to a denervated and lax sphincteric urethra. In this latter group the upper urinary tract is ordinarily normal and infection is not a problem.

Incontinence of various degrees, usually continuous dribbling, is the rule in both of these broad categories. With minimal neurological deficit urinary continence may be associated with only subtle symptoms of straining to urinate and occasional episodes of urgency. For the purposes of definition, a somatic nerve lesion should always be identifiable in making this diagnosis. In this regard, minimal areas of heel and perianal sensory loss, obtunded anal or bulbocavernosus reflex, or electromyographic evidence of perineal neurological deficit should be carefully assessed to corroborate the underlying nature of the lesion.

The "suspect" neurogenic bladder, manifested largely by hypotonia and sometimes assumed to be due to aganglionosis or defects in the neuromuscular transmission system of the hypogastric plexus, does not have an established place in this classification on our present level of knowledge. The most frequently observed type of lower motor-neuron, unbalanced, neurogenic bladder secondary to dysrhaphia is the hypertrophied type showing a thickened vesical neck on voiding cystourethrography, multiple diverticula, and frequently ureteral reflux. This state of affairs, particularly in girls, is associated with refractory urinary tract infection (Fig. 58).

The histological mural changes in the detrusor muscle are as widely varied as its defective innervation and unpredictable function. In a group of biopsies examined in the course of this study from several areas of the bladder, all of the changes seen in hypertrophy, long-

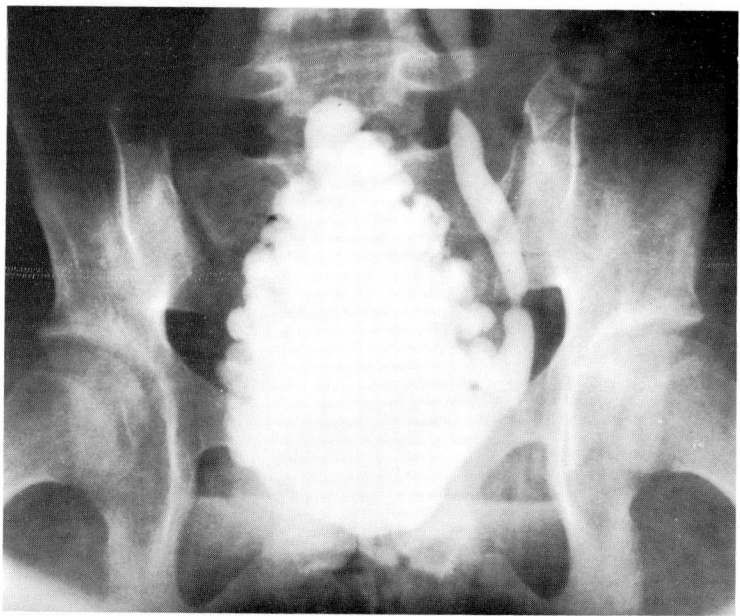

FIG. 58. Attempted voiding cystourethrogram to show hypertrophied and "functionally" obstructed neurogenic bladder, associated with myelomeningocele in 8-year-old girl. Diverticula and left ureteral reflux are prominent features here. Note lack of funnelling of the vesical neck.

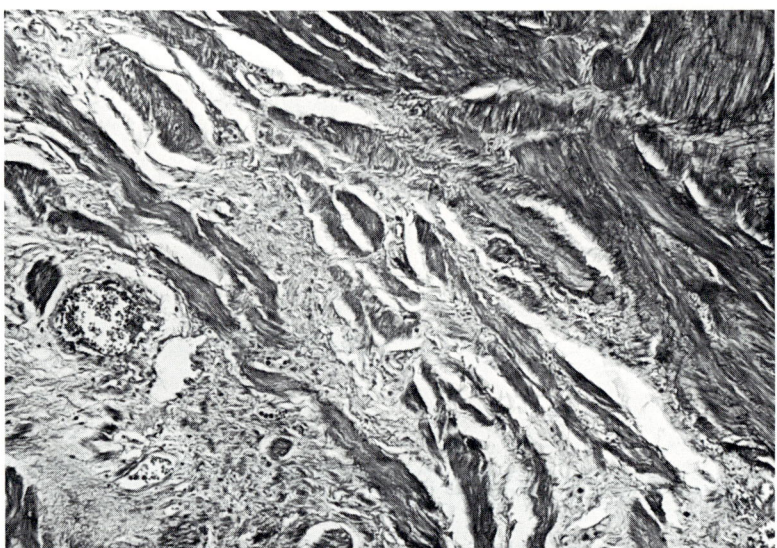

FIG. 59. Photomicrograph of mural structure of neurogenic bladder secondary to myelomeningocele in a 3-year old boy. Note area of smooth muscle bundle hypertrophy with elastic fiber prominence (upper right). Adjacent areas of fibroelastosis and sparse muscle fascicles (lower left). Verhoeff-van Gieson stain. Original magnification X100.

standing obstruction, dysplasia and "fibroelastosis" could be demonstrated. In addition, inflammatory changes in the tunica propria and the mucosa add further confusion to the histological appearance. A single overall feature, frequently observed, was the association of immediately adjacent areas of marked hypertrophy of smooth-muscle bundles, showing normal organization, but with increased numbers of elastic fibers, and areas showing dense fibrosis with small muscle bundles containing only a few thin and erratically distributed smooth-muscle cells (Fig. 59).

In the fibrotic regions collagen and elastin are densely associated, giving the appearance of "fibroelastosis." Whether these represent primary areas of denervated muscle-bundle complexes adjacent to normal and/or hypertrophied ones, or merely a secondary pressure phenomenon manifested by diverticulum formation, is impossible to say. Normal nerves and some ganglia could be identified in the adventitia. From this biopsy material it is not possible to make any statement as to the relative *number* of ganglion cells or nerves present.

From a functional standpoint, the massive incoordination of the bladder and sphincteric musculature and secondary changes of infection and fibroelastosis create a difficult complex to treat surgically with any anticipation of success. For this reason, early urinary diversion has become increasingly popular in recent years.[477] By applying a knowledge of the normal function in the structure of the bladder, it may be possible, in many cases with more minor involvement of the sacral cord, to augment whatever contractility and sphincteric function exists by a planned increase in the expulsive muscular elements combined with judicious weakening of the retentive ones. It would also seem wise to defer procedures for permanent urinary diversion until the functional capacity of the neurogenic bladder can be assessed adequately. Perhaps this is not entirely possible until the age of five or six years.

Inflammatory Obstruction

Urethral obstruction due solely to urinary tract infection is probably largely transient. In the female child with urethritis some degree of smooth-muscle dysfunction may be induced by infection alone. This often accounts for the apparently abnormal voiding urethrograms obtained during episodes of infection. Repetition of the examination following control of the infection has shown that the urethra returns to its normal configuration.[458]

In the studies of Young, Anderson and King[558] on the behavior of ascendent Lipiodol in the bladder, floating Lipiodol was retained in the bladders of some children during acute infections for periods of longer than 72 hours. Subsequent Lipiodol studies, when the children were uninfected, showed prompt evacuation of the ascendent Lipiodol within 24 hours. Involuntary smooth-muscle spasm secondary to tissue inflammatory response might well account for these findings.

Urethral Meatal Stenosis

Urethral meatal scarring and stenosis in the male infant secondary to urinary dermatitis with ulceration is a well-known cause of meatal obstruction, and easily diagnosed. Urethral meatal stenosis in girls has a different basis and is quite significant as a cause of recurrent lower urinary tract infection. This "distal urethral stenosis," as it has been aptly called by Lyon and Smith[326] and Lyon and Tanagho,[327] is caused by varying degrees of rigidity of the normally dense collagenous confluence of the hymenal ring with the entire posterior (dorsal) lip of the urethral meatus, rather than by a specific decrease in its caliber.

In infant girls the urethral meatus is often obscured by soft folds of hymenal mucosa. This is of not great significance; nor are minor variations in urethral caliber. It is the excessive rigidity of the meatus, which may extend into the lumen for several millimeters, which leads to the deformed ballooning of the immature, softly muscled, proximal sphincteric urethra during urination. It seems probable that this hydrodynamically unfavorable configuration produces increased turbulent countercurrents for transport of bacteria into the bladder.

Inflammatory edema and necrosis of prolapsed urethral mucosa in infant girls is an obvious mechanical type of obstruction. This usually produces an acute but partial outflow obstruction. The diagnosis is evident upon simple inspection.

Other causes of urethral obstruction include prolapsing ureterocele[142] and extrinsic lesions exerting pressure against the base of the bladder, vesical neck or sphincteric urethra. These include hydromucocolpos, pelvic masses, tumors and abscesses, as well as the feces-filled rectum.

Tumor

Symptoms of urinary obstruction may be the presenting complaint in a child with embryonic sarcoma arising from the mesenchyme of the urogenital sinus. These tumors ordinarily contain muscular elements and various degrees of attempted formation of striations among the myofibrils. The term *rhabdomyosarcoma* suits the lesion best.[540,544]

This tumor, affecting male children more frequently than females, usually occurs in the first four years of life. Since it originates from the urogenital sinus, it has been characterized as sarcoma of the prostate, sarcoma of the vagina or as sarcoma of the bladder (sarcoma botryoides). Involvement of the bladder and surrounding tissues may be extensive. The sphincteric urethra is almost invariably involved in submucosal extensions of the tumor. The absolute incidence of these tumors is difficult to determine. Fourteen cases have been seen by Williams,[544] of whom nine have survived at least three years following radical surgery. This is the largest single series of cases reported.

Most of the reports in the literature are of individual or, at most, three or four cases.[49,81,349,532,283,359] Rhabdomyosarcoma is an extremely malignant tumor and the associated complications of infection, hypertrophy of the bladder and gradual upper-tract damage are usually telescoped into the brief survival period of the child. Classical signs of chronic obstruction are usually absent.

Other malignant tumors of the lower urinary tract, even more rare, are neurofibromas associated with other distant lesions.[501,112] A family history of this disease and the associated stigmata of neurofibromatosis in the patient help in making the diagnosis.

Hemangiomas, frequently with wide involvement of the surrounding pelvic organs, may involve the bladder and urethra. However, these are not usually obstructive.

V

Management

Diagnosis

From a physiopathological study such as this, it can be seen that there is a considerable degree of overlapping among the pathological obstructive changes within the lower urinary tract. The primarily obstructing lesion, although responsible as a first cause for secondary changes, may not be the most severe threat to the infant. Clinical classification is, therefore, difficult.

The urologist cannot expect a single cause to produce a single condition which can always be easily corrected by one surgical procedure or course of antibacterial therapy. It is probably more exact, when reasoning through the diagnosis and planning treatment, to consider the intimate histological structure and composite function of the affected structures in the individual child than to attempt to manage an arbitrary class or degree of obstruction with some standard or popular method of treatment. For this reason, I should like to stress only general principles of diagnosis and treatment of the child with lower urinary tract obstruction and indicate those which seem to promise the greatest benefit.

The diagnostic management of the child with urinary obstruction begins with history and observation, followed by examination. The history is often meager. The younger the child, the fewer the clues. Classical symptoms of urinary tract disease in the adult are rarely seen in children under the age of 10. The urologist must many times be content with the incidental finding of pyuria by the pediatrician, an increased odor, or a trace of pink urine on the diaper.

During the course of the urologist's initial examination, the child can be observed and the history taken from the parent at the same time. The pediatric urologist must be aware of the anatomical and physiological variations of the urinary tract and their manifestations in the symptoms and signs which he is seeking. He must ferret out variations in the normal patterns of physiology and anatomy by his questions, in order quickly to compare them with his special knowledge of normal urinary structure and function in the child.

It is important to remember that during the first day of life urinary output is low due to low fluid intake, low blood pressure and low renal blood flow. During the first year of life, the child excretes roughly two-thirds of its fluid intake. The newborn infant may urinate as often as 15 to 20 times during a 24-hour period, but with fluid loss in vomiting or diarrhea the urinary output may be reduced to 30 to 60 ml per day. The specific gravity of the urine is low during the first year of life due to the relative inability of the renal tubules to concentrate the filtrate to any great degree. Micturition occurs largely in a reflex manner at birth and until the age of two years, by which time the child is usually dry during the day with only an occasional accident. By the age of four, children are ordinarily dry day and night; however, there may be temporary regressions to nocturnal enuresis.

Pain, as a symptom of urinary tract disease in children, is not usually a chief complaint; nor are frequency and dysuria. Pain is manifested in infants by aimless activity, kicking or crying, and, in the case of bladder spasm or ureteral colic, may be characterized by intermittency which can be determined by close observation. In children under the age of five or six, abdominal and flank pain is usually localized to the umbilicus; the child recognizes this as the only salient landmark on its vast abdominal expanse. Fever, convulsions, vomiting and gastrointestinal symptoms are more important indications of obstructive uropathy than is pain.

Hematuria, when present, is a red flag not easily overlooked by the mother. Hematuria in the male is most frequently related to small meatal ulcers, crystalluria or urinary tract infection. Hematuria due to infection is less common in children than in adults. Total, gross, painless hematuria more frequently suggests acute glomerulonephritis in children than it does either tumor or infection. Red urine can be produced by an intracellular pigment in beets and by certain food colorings.

Failure of normal growth may be related to urinary tract disease on the basis of uremia or chronic infection with attendant anemia.

Pyuria may be noted by the mother as a persistent cloudiness of the urine, but is usually overlooked unless a specimen is obtained specifically for examination by the physician. Cloudy urine may be due to leukocytes or bacteria, but is frequently due to crystals. The mother will often notice increased odor to the urine; this is indicative of urinary tract infection.

Urinary frequency in older children may be due to local causes as well as to urinary tract infection. Pinworms, producing a vaginitis or ammoniacal dermatitis involving the labia, can cause frequency and local pain.

Urgency in children is manifested by "wetting."

Incontinence is not a particularly descriptive term for use in evaluating urinary symptoms in children, although it does occur in certain circumstances, particularly with neurogenic bladders secondary to lower motor-neuron lesions where there is usually constant urinary dribbling. This may represent overflow incontinence accompanied by a large amount of residual urine, or it may be due to flaccid paralysis of the sphincteric urethra associated with a perennially collapsed bladder.

In examination of the child's abdomen, a suprapubic midline mass will usually represent the bladder. This may present some confusion, as the child's bladder is more of an intra-abdominal organ and relatively larger than it is in the adult. With urination, the mass may completely disappear. If it remains, it may indicate the presence of a large amount of residual urine in a greatly thickened and hypertrophied bladder. Palpable masses in the lumbar quadrant suggest either cystic disease, hydronephrosis or renal neoplasm. Hydronephrotic kidneys, although occasionally percussible, are difficult to palpate.

Pneumaturia, or the passage of meconium in the urine, usually calls attention to a congenital rectourethral or rectovesical fistula. These fistulae are usually associated with either imperforate anus or one of the cloacal variations and the abnormality will be evident upon examination of the perineum and with endoscopy.

In children under two years, three positive historical features can be easily determined which indicate a normal urinary pattern: (1) There should be a good, full urinary stream with a sharp beginning and sharp end-point; (2) there should be no straining associated with micturition; and (3) dry periods should be observed from birth.

In the general examination of the child, associated anomalies or developmental deformities should be assessed. Abnormalities of the urinary tract can be associated with cardiovascular and musculoskeletal defects. Defects in the sacral spine can sometimes be palpated easily. The external genitalia should be carefully inspected. The presence of normal epididymides and vasa deferentia in males can always be verified, even in the youngest infant. Perineal sensation is easily determined, as is anal sphincter tone. Rectal examination should always be performed.

Diagnostic Investigation

No single diagnostic study may be applied in every case, nor is any invariably correct surgical procedure indicated for all cases of a given class of congenital obstructive disease. The most important diagnostic laboratory procedures are, in the order of their importance: (1) measurement of serum concentrations of creatinine, blood urea nitrogen and electrolytes, followed by (2) intravenous urography with voiding cystourethrography. There are specific conditions, as in the infant with severely progressive renal failure, in which intravenous urography cannot be performed satisfactorily and cystography with reflux pyelography, or even percutaneous "antegrade" pyelography, must be substituted in order to visualize the upper urinary tract.

Renal scanning with radioactive isotope-labelled Hippuran in the neonate may be of considerable value in differentiating massive hydronephrosis from renal agenesis or hypoplasia.

Cystography and voiding cystourethrography, in which the contour and function of the sphincteric urethra can be made out, is probably a more important study than cystoscopy in the infant. The potential of the voiding cystourethrogram includes demonstration of ureteral reflux, variations in the mural configuration and thickness of the bladder wall, sites of obstruction within the sphincteric urethra or distal urethra and estimates of persistent residual urine. This latter can be more accurately determined by the addition of ascendant Lipiodol (10%) to instilled contrast medium and the subsequent demonstration of its persistence or absence on delayed films.[558]

With special equipment, intravesical pressure tracings and estimates of urethral resistance can be combined with voiding cystourethrography. Cineradiography applied to the voiding cystourethrogram provides a dynamic record of a single urination. This study has been useful in establishing normal flow rates and pressure patterns and their correlation with the radiographic appearance of the voided bladder urine. Clinically, the voiding cystourethrogram, with several single films taken of the most important events during urination, probably offers as much useful information as these more highly sophisticated, and pro re nata more cumbersome, studies. The voiding cystourethrogram in the infant or child performed at the close of excretory urography provides an almost complete urographic study and, when it has been well performed, weighs heavily in the diagnostic balance. In evaluating the voiding cystourethrogram, the opacified urine within the lumen must be regarded as merely a negative image of the surrounding anatomical structures. It is the structure of the sphincteric urethra and its functional disturbances which must be estimated—not the flow of the column of urine.

Residual urine as an indication of lower urinary tract obstruction has long been regarded not only as an important diagnostic sign but as a potential reservoir for chronic infection once bacterial growth becomes established. It is now abundantly clear that all measured bladder residuum after voiding is not necessarily retained in the bladder. A portion of this may represent refluxed ureteral urine which has secondarily returned to the bladder following urination. In some cases, all of the measured bladder residual represents ureteral reflux.[230,126,193,382]

Cinecystourethrography is probably the single most informative demonstration of the actual nature of the residual urine in any given case. It is important to make a distinction between vesical residual urine alone and that due to reflux. *Ureteral residual urine* is dependent upon incompetence of the ureterovesical junctions, from whatever cause. *Vesical residual urine*, on the other hand, is related to dysfunction of the detrusor muscle based on either obstruction of the sphincteric urethra or incomplete contraction of the detrusor itself. It is uncommon to find residual urine in male patients with distal urethral strictures or in children with meatal stenosis.

As a diagnostic sign of detrusor decompensation, the measurement of residual urine is perhaps comparable to the finding of elevated central venous pressure or basilar rales as indicative of cardiac failure. In adults, it constitutes mainly corroborative evidence and is rarely used alone as an indication of vesical-neck obstruction, except in neurogenic dysfunction of the bladder.

The actual volume of residual urine is not as important as its persistence. It is not paramount to know the extent to which the detrusor mechanism is decompensated; the fact that it is decompensated *at all* is the significant point.

Ascendant Lipiodol instillation, although requiring catheterization, has the advantage of requiring only a single procedure of this type, subsequent information being obtained and documented radiographically. Refluxed Lipiodol droplets have sometimes been noted in the renal collecting systems on delayed films, when no reflux could be demonstrated by voiding cystourethrography. The physician can feel a definite security if all of the Lipiodol is absent at the end of 24 hours. In some children an immediate postvoiding film will show absence of the oil, in which case the study is complete. However, it is desirable to allow a child to engage in several leisurely urinations over a 24-hour period, without having to void on the spot (Fig. 60).

Endoscopy in infants and children should be regarded in a different light than cystoscopy in the adult. A limited number of conditions can be diagnosed *only* by direct cystoscopic examination. These include: urachal cysts, ectopic ureteral or fistulous orifices, and possibly radiolucent foreign bodies which may not be visualized with radiographic studies.

Cystourethroscopy in both male and female infants and children is a largely confirmatory study. In many cases endoscopic surgical procedures can be anticipated in advance and carried out at the same time as the examination. In only rare instances should cystourethroscopy be carried out in children without anesthesia. The procedure is not only uncomfortable and frightening to a child but, more important, the examination is often incomplete; brief impressions cannot be verified, unexpected lesions cannot be biopsied, plical folds

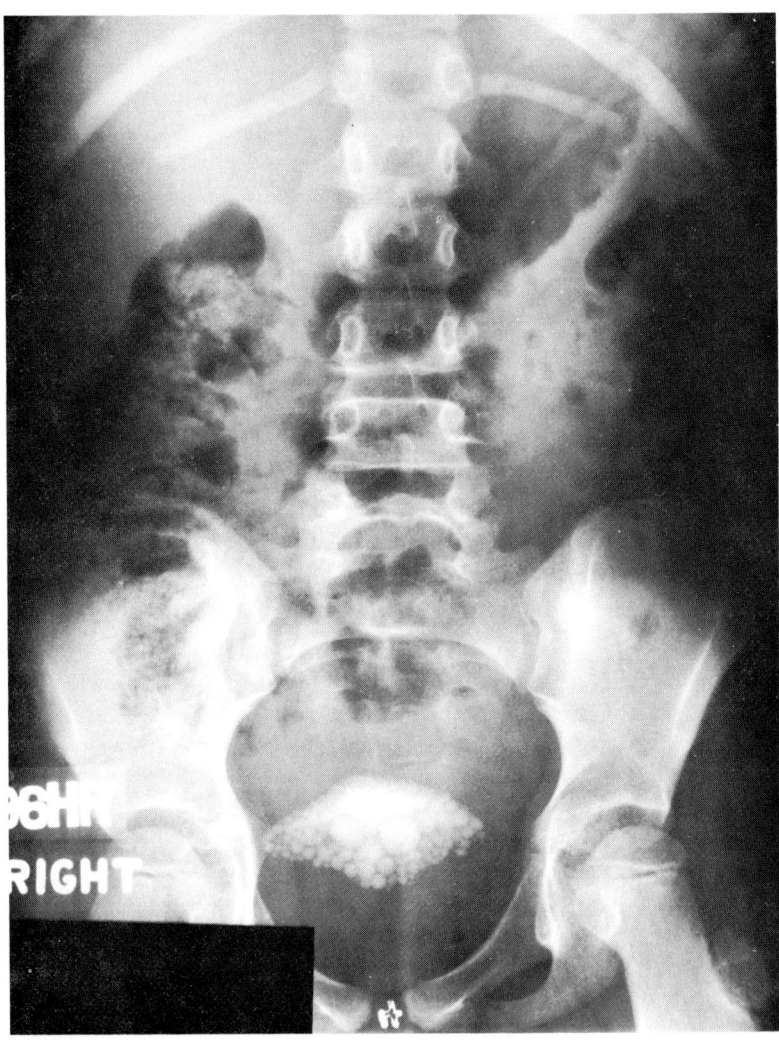

FIG. 60. Case J.O. Persistent residual urine demonstrated by the presence of ascendant Lipiodol at 96 hours. No evidence of reflux of Lipiodol to either kidney.

cannot be destroyed with electrocoagulation, nor can the urethra be dilated or meatotomy performed.

Endoscopy must therefore be regarded as a full-scale surgical procedure in the child, no matter how confident the urologist is of his skill or the apparent simplicity of the procedure. It is true that endoscopy may not reveal positive findings, and that the examination will not confirm questionable findings of previous radiological and clinical examinations. This is in a sense a negative triumph—and in such cases an unnecessary examination.

Cystoscopy should not be considered a mandatory examination for every child referred to the urologist. The decision to proceed with endoscopy should be awarded the same consideration as a decision to proceed with any surgical procedure. It should be carried out only when preliminary studies indicate a reasonable possibility that the diagnosis and treatment will be distinctly furthered by the examination.

Special radiological studies are often combined with endoscopy and can be quite valuable. Retrograde urethrography or urogenital sinus radiography is probably best carried out by the urologist. It may be necessary to identify small vaginal orifices endoscopically and catheterize them by this method in intersexes or in children with ambiguous genitalia.

Transurethral resection of valves, vesical neck or ureteroceles (if necessary, inserting the instrument through a perineal urethrostomy) can be carried out under the same anesthetic, if planned in advance.

The sequence of study and treatment of the child is, then, in logical order:

1. History
2. Observation
3. Examination
4. Urinalysis
5. Estimation of renal function and blood studies, including electrolytes, when indicated
6. Excretory urography, with voiding cystourethrography, in a combined examination
7. Voiding cystourethrography as a separate study following instillation of the contrast material by catheter. (It is at this point that the more sophisticated variations, such as cinecystometrography and measurements of exit pressures for calculating urethral resistance, can be carried out.)
8. Endoscopy and endoscopic surgery
9. Surgery or medical management

Treatment

In treatment, the principal aim is to establish a continent urinary bladder which can empty itself completely and maintain a sterile urine.

Modest though this requirement may seem, it is sometimes impossible.

Surgical procedures should be directed at the elimination of residual urine, both within the bladder and in the ureters. In pursuing this end based upon anatomical and physiological principles, the concept of *balance* is the surgical guide. Once we know the nature of the basic obstructive phenomenon and the extent of its secondary damaging effects, we are in a position to plan a surgical program.

The *sphincteric urethra can be weakened* by dividing the detrusor loop ventrally, or by Y-V vesicourethroplasty (Figs. 61, 62).[559,196,333,115,187,194] The *ureterovesical junctions can be reconstructed* quite successfully to prevent reflux.[187,406,24,240,392,186] *Reduction cystoplasty* can be used, as a somewhat crude method, to decrease the capacity of the bladder. The full potential of increasing the expulsive force of the bladder has not been explored. Vesical plication or detrusor imbrication in combination with vesicourethroplasty has not been investigated fully. *Seromuscular grafts of bowel wall* have not been given sufficient clinical trial. Further possibilities to attain a balanced bladder include selective weakening of particular muscle groups in the detrusor, particularly *division of the heavy posterior longitudinal bundle* or resection of the anterior longitudinal muscle bundle above the vesical neck to prevent anterior funnelling during voiding. This might be considered as an operation for alleviating minor degrees of incontinence.

There are possibilities of *neuromuscular blockade or stimulation* of the bladder with drugs, in conjunction with surgical procedures, which might prove productive. Pudendal block or resection of the pudendal nerves has been used in neurogenic bladders in this manner to reduce sphincteric resistance due to spasticity of the perineal striated musculature. The ultimate in balance would probably be the construction of a functional smooth-muscle sphincter from transplanted smooth muscle of the detrusor.

Surgical attempts at producing a balanced bladder in these varying pathological conditions can never be more than approximations. Growth, hypertrophy and training fortunately assist the child in the finer tuning of the surgical result.

Ideally, following successful reconstructive surgery, a single course of an appropriate antibacterial agent should sterilize the urine and, in the absence of residual urine, the urinary tract should be able to maintain itself in this condition and function normally. Unfortunately,

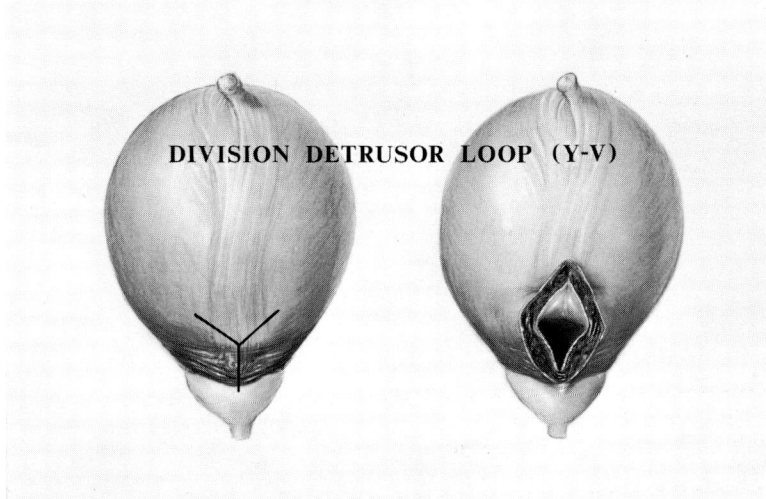

FIG. 61. Drawing to indicate the functional basis of Y-V vesicourethroplasty. This consists merely of dividing the detrusor loop and interposing anterior longitudinal bundle fibers to prevent its normal arcuate contractile function as the anterior half of the internal sphincter.

this is not always the case. Despite adequate surgical procedures, many of these conditions cannot be corrected because of irreparable fibrosis or congenital absence of essential structures. We must sometimes compromise and accept partial continence, small amounts of residual urine and chronic infection.

Further Considerations

When all reasonable surgical procedures have been carried out in attempting to achieve balance of the lower urinary tract, and the child still maintains residual urine with uncontrolled infection, the patient must be managed with a prolonged medical regimen. The guide for the urologist, here, is the word "patience." In many cases, conservative medical management must be carried out until the child attains puberty and, in some, the sequelae of childhood urinary tract damage must be followed throughout the patient's adult life. Some extremely important positive factors peculiar to the child reinforce the physician's patience. The first is normal growth and maturation. This applies to the urethral and trigonal epithelium and the estrogen influence exerted

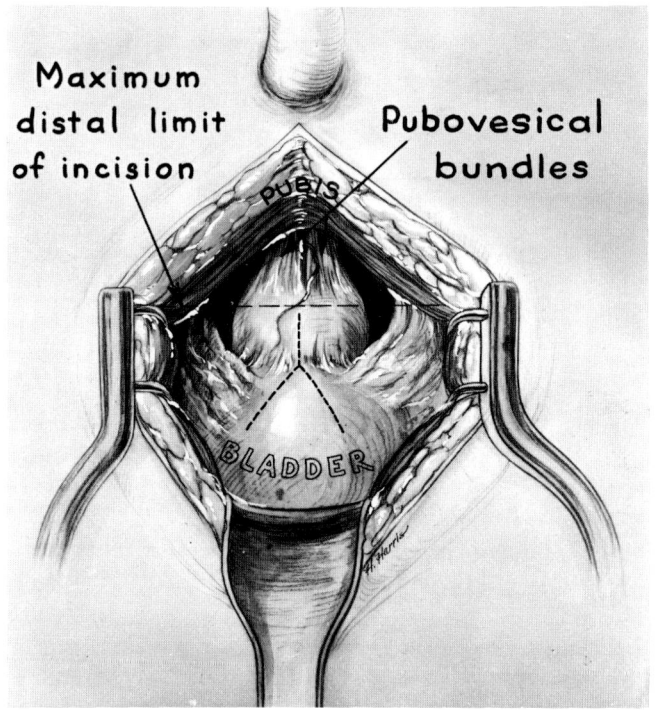

FIG. 62. See legend on facing page.

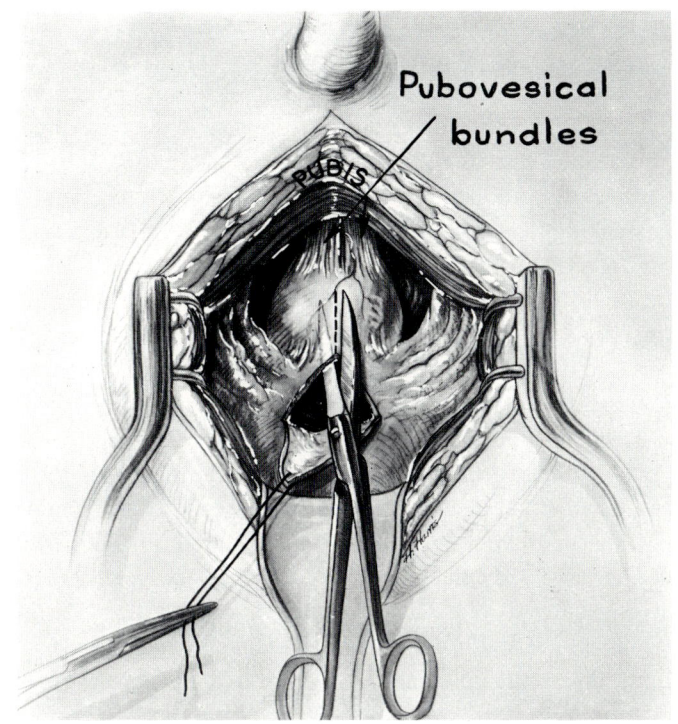

C

FIG. 62. Semidiagrammatic drawings of the Y-V type of vesicourethroplasty. The incision is outlined in *A*. It will be noted that the distal limb of the Y is kept well above the pubovesical bundles. *B*, Hooked blade is used to make the initial V. *C*, Detrusor loops are divided with the scissors.

upon it by the menarche in girls, to the increased maturation of the detrusor muscle and ureterovesical junctions particularly,[241] and to normal growth of the kidney, which is not complete until the ages of 15 to 17. The second comforting factor is anticipated hypertrophy—both the hypertrophy of the smooth musculature of the entire urinary tract and the responsive hypertrophy of a single kidney, or even a portion of one, challenged by severe damage to its mate. A third factor, though less predictable, is the child's increasing cooperation and gradual molding of urinary habit patterns.

The basis of medical management is, of course, antibacterial therapy and an increased fluid intake to produce an increased volume of urine, necessitating frequent voidings. There is no specific antibacterial maintenance regimen which can be universally recommended for general management. The subject of urinary tract infection is beyond the scope of this monograph and has been intensively studied by others. Striking advances continue to be made in the control of bacterial infection.

The broad principles here are several. Ninety percent of urinary tract infections are due to Gram-negative bacilli and, accordingly, are responsive to antibacterial drugs with that particular spectrum. The least toxic and best tolerated antibacterial medication, in the smallest dosage commensurate with control of recurrences of pyelonephritis, is the drug of choice. Bacterial infection of the kidney is the major threat to its function and to the patient's survival. Recurrent cystitis is not a fatal or progressive disease and is significant only in that it provides an easily available pool of bacteria for recurrent pyelonephritis.

Progressive variations in the size of each kidney with growth should not invariably be regarded as progressive pyelonephritic damage to the smaller of the two kidneys. This appearance can be produced by compensatory hypertrophy of the normal kidney. Variation in renal sizes may represent "growth lag" of the previously damaged and fibrotic kidney, or even a lack of full potential growth due to dysplastic changes within the lagging kidney.

Close observation is the most important function of the patient urologist. This does not necessarily mean continuous instrumentation, cystoscopy, or repeated urography and cinecystourethrography. Repeated urethral dilatations in the female child are more a manifestation of an anxious urologist than of a progressively contracting urethra. The potential of local damage to the delicate sphincteric urethra by repeated dilations seems far greater than the danger of the disease. Repeated cystoscopies with varying findings of cystitis cystica, erythema of the trigone, urethral edema or varying appearances of the ureteral orifices over the years are interesting as observations, but perhaps not particularly valuable to the patient as far as therapy is concerned. Repeated intravenous urograms at short intervals are unlikely to disclose any new information if the initial studies have been carefully carried out. It is important, however, to repeat renal function studies at intervals; occasionally a "short series" intravenous urogram can be obtained in which no more than three or four films need to be made.

Yearly evaluations should be carried out in children with complicated obstructive urological problems. On each occasion these should be approached as fresh cases, with all previously planned surgical procedures, new techniques in management, and advances in antibacterial management taken into account.

As part of the management program, *training*, particularly in female children, can be most important. Children under the age of two are unable to accomplish double or triple voiding. Shortly after the child is capable of urinating at will, she can be taught to double void—with varying degrees of success, to be sure. Vaginal reflux of voided urine in little girls is more frequent than previously realized; little girls should be taught to aid vaginal drainage following urination by remaining a few minutes more on the toilet with their legs widely spread, and drying the vulva should be made more than a ritual. The need for perineal hygiene is perhaps too obvious to mention. It should be remembered that soap is irritating to the vaginal mucosa and its effects are more likely to stimulate resistance to washing the vulva than to encourage it. Warm water squeezed from a cotton ball over the vulva is perhaps equally effective.

It is possible to establish a pattern of increased fluid intake and frequent conscious voidings in girls who are prone to infection, and even to train them to arise several times at night to urinate, should this be necessary. Gradual transference of the entire responsibility for bladder function from the parent to the young child is most important, and is also the key to disturbed behavior patterns manifested by enuresis in the child with a perfectly normal urinary tract.

Permanent urinary diversion in the child, although an unquestionably impressive and dramatic surgical procedure, is not the *cure* of urinary tract obstruction in any sense of the word. Quite the reverse, it is a confession of failure in the face of insurmountable disease, and is a decision on the part of the surgeon and parents to preserve a sort of half-life for the child rather than to accept the alternatives. Permanent nephrostomy in infants and children has been, in my experience, a delayed death warrant, exceedingly difficult to manage and worthy of all attempts at other substitutes, including anastomosis of the renal pelvis to isolated loops of ileum, or renal transplantation.

In the child with progressive hydronephrosis, uncontrollable infection and progressive pyelonephritis, ileal-loop urinary diversion has proven to be a most satisfactory procedure, despite its surgical complications. It is well to remember that, following uretero-ileal diversion, there is no possibility of later salvage of the sacrificed lower urinary tract. This type of diversion should be classed as a desperate surgical operation designed for the preservation of life, after all hope of growth, compensatory hypertrophy and maturation has been abandoned.

Occasionally, large, dilated ureters with adequate peristalsis will permit ureteroureterocutaneous anastomosis to achieve the same result as permanent ileal-loop urinary diversion. If urine is to be collected in a bag, the methods and sites of application are only technical considerations in the individual case.

Permanent urinary diversion for lesions of the lower urinary tract which are not amenable to reconstruction, such as exstrophy, persistent urogenital sinus and third-degree epispadias with absence of the sphincteric urethra, can be managed by ureteral transplantation to an isolated rectal pouch, with the proximal loop of sigmoid colon brought out through the anal sphincter adjacent to the rectal urinary stoma as in the Heitz-Boyer-Hovelacque or Gersuny procedures. This can be carried out only in the child with a well-functioning anal sphincter. Currently, this procedure for urinary diversion appears to offer many advantages, including a modest separation of the urinary and fecal streams and the absence of an external urinary collection device. The operation of ureterosigmoidostomy for permanent urinary diversion in children should be seriously reconsidered now that there are available improved methods of sterilizing the bowel preoperatively which maintain a relative bacteria-free area of healing at the anastomosis site for several days. In addition, long-term, relatively nontoxic antibacterial therapy of urinary tract infection can now be carried out more effectively than in the past.

Indiscriminate early ileal-loop urinary diversion in children with neurogenic bladders secondary to myelomeningocele carried out at very early ages is not acceptable. One must consider that the child has 13 to 15 years of life prior to puberty during which the full potential of the detrusor, substitutive neuromuscular systems and the growth potential of the kidney can be realized. Our basic knowledge of the normal anatomy and function of the neuromuscular system in the urinary tract is sketchy at present but may improve sufficiently to offer other alternatives. The exact nature of the neuromuscular defects in the random lesions affecting the cauda equina and sacral cord in dysrhaphia is notoriously obscure. It seems that the correct approach at this time in children with these defects should be conservative; permanent urinary diversion is indicated only for reasons of progressive renal failure and uncontrollable upper-urinary tract infection, as it is for other severe urinary obstructive disease in children.

The term *management* means more than simply guiding the patient. The physician, too, must manage his enthusiasms and aspirations, his occasional paralysis of action by considerations, his reasonable sense of urgency, which threatens to become haste, and, most dangerous of all, his scientific convictions. These impulses are the surgeon's constant companions, but they cannot be allowed to distort crucial observations, judgments or procedures to the detriment of the patient. What, then, is a safe base for pursuing the immediate case at hand? In this monograph I hope to have indicated a composite outline of the underlying anatomical and physiological processes bearing upon lower urinary tract obstruction in childhood.

I would say: Revere the anatomy to its most minute level, and its function to the last pliant contraction of the smooth-muscle walls. Pathological changes within these balanced structures must be minutely identified and specifically destroyed or corrected, with the single aim of restoring or approximating normal function.

It is with honest humility but no pride that we must admit our inability to construct an adequate mechanical substitute for the urethral sphincter, although this may be an ultimate possibility. Be that as it may, its effective function over a life span of seventy years will have to accomplish the purpose which the normal urinary tract accomplishes without notice or applause.

The pediatric urological surgeon of today is best advised to restore normal structure and function using the materials at hand, which, after all, were very well designed.

VI
Bibliography

1. Albarran, J.: In Poirier et Charpy: *Triaté d'Anatomie Humaine,* Tome 5:257. Paris, Masson et Cie, 1923.
2. Alesio, C. and Pisani, L.: *La Malattia del Collo Vesicale.* Torino, 1931.
3. Alken, C. E.: *Leitfadender Urologie,* S. 137. Stuttgart, 1955.
4. Ambrose, S. S. and Nicolson, W. P.: The causes of vesicoureteral reflux in children. J. Urol. 87:688-694, 1962.
5. Ambrose, S. S. and Nicolson, W. P.: Vesicoureteral reflux secondary to anomalies of the ureterovesical junction: Management and results. J. Urol. 87:695-700, 1962.
6. Andreassen, M.: Vesical neck obstruction in children. Acta Chir. Scand. 105:398-406, 1953.
7. Arbuckle, L. D., Jr. and Paquin, A. J., Jr.: Urinary outflow tract resistance in normal human females. Invest. Urol. 1:216-228, 1963.
8. Arey, L. B.: *Developmental Anatomy.* Philadelphia, W. B. Saunders, 1941.
9. Badenoch, A. W.: Congenital obstruction of the bladder neck. Ann. Roy. Coll. Surg. Eng. 4:295-307, 1949.
10. Baker, R., Tehan, T. and Kelly, K.: Observations on 100 children with bladder neck obstruction. J. Urol. 84:334-339, 1960.
11. Baldridge, R. R.: A case of congenital hypertrophy of the verumontanum. New Eng. J. Med. 213:46-49, 1935.
12. Barkow, H. C.: *Anatomische Untersuchunger über die Harnblase des Menschen.* Breslau, F. Hirt, 1858.
13. Barrie, H. J. and Simms, D. C.: Hydronephrosis resulting from obstruction of the urethra by a polyp of verumontanum. Amer. J. Clin. Path. 36:356-361, 1961.
14. Basmajian, J. V. and Spring, W. B.: Electromyography of the male (voluntary) sphincter urethrae. Anat. Rec. 121:388, 1955.
15. Bazy, M.: Oblitération de l'urètre par une valvule congénitale en forme de diaphragme.—Résection.—Guérison. Bull. Soc. Chir. Paris 29:32-48, 1903.
16. Beer, E.: Chronic retention of urine in children. J.A.M.A. 65:1709-1712, 1915.
17. Beer, E.: Chronic retention of urine in young boys due to obstruction at neck of bladder. Ann. Surg. 79:264-269, 1924.

18. Bell, C.: *A Treatise on the Disease of the Urethra, Vesica Urinaria, Prostate and Rectum.* London, Longman, 1820.
19. Bengmark, S.: The occurrence of degeneration phenomena during the process of separation of the primitive ureter from the wolffian duct. Urol. Int. 8:117-125, 1959.
20. Benjamin, J. A., Joint, F. T., Ramsay, G. H., Watson, J. S., Weinberg, S. and Scott, W. E.: Cinéfluorographic studies of bladder and urethral function. J. Urol. 73:525-535, 1955.
21. Bergman, R. A.: Intercellular bridges in smooth muscle. Bull. Hopkins Hosp. 102:195-202, 1958.
22. Bevans, M.: Changes in the musculature of the gastrointestinal tract and in the myocardium in progressive muscular dystrophy. Arch. Path. 40:225-238, 1945.
23. Biro, J.: Biochemical composition of the vesical musculature. In *Internationale Konferenz für Urologie* (November 1962). Akadémial Kiado., Budapest, 1964.
24. Bischoff, P.: Megaureter. Brit. J. Urol. 29:416-423, 1957.
25. Blechschmidt, E.: *The Stages of Human Development before Birth: An Introduction to Human Embryology.* Philadelphia, W. B. Saunders, 1961.
26. Bloomfield, A. and Frazer, J. E.: The development of the lower end of the vagina. J. Anat. 62:9-32, 1927.
27. Bodian, M.: Some observations on the pathology of congenital idiopathic bladder neck obstruction (Marion's disease). Brit. J. Urol. 29:393-398, 1957.
28. Bonnet, P.: Cited by Pagano, F.: Le valvole congenite dell'uretra. Urologia 16 (Suppl.):64-106, 1965.
29. Bonney, V.: On diurnal incontinence of urine in women. J. Obstet. Gynaec. Brit. Emp. 30:358-365, 1923.
30. Bonnin, N. J.: Plastic reconstruction of the bladder neck and prostatectomy: An operation suitable for all types of non-malignant bladder neck obstructions. Aust. New Zeal. J. Surg. 27:161-173, 1957-1958.
31. Bonnin, N. J.: Thoughts on sphincteric function and comments on management of bladder outlet obstruction in the female. Brit. J. Urol. 41:465-473, 1969.
32. Borm, D. and Clausen E.: Die Blasensphinktersklerose. Bruns Beitr. Klin. Chir. 4:447-468, 1963.
33. Bors, E.: Effect of electrical stimulation of the pudendal nerves on the vesical neck: its significance for the function of cord bladders: a preliminary report. J. Urol. 67:925-935, 1952.
34. Bors, E., Comarr, A. E. and Reingold, I. M.: Striated muscle fibers of the vesical neck. J. Urol. 72:191-196, 1954.
35. Bors, E., Ma, K. T. and Parker, R. B.: Observations on some modalities of bladder sensation. J. Urol. 76:566-575, 1956.
36. Bors, E. and Blinn, K.: Spinal reflex activity from the vesical mucosa in paraplegic patients. Arch. Neurol. Psychiat. 78:339-354, 1957.
37. Bors, E.: Neurogenic bladder. Urol. Survey, 7:177-250, 1957.
38. Bourne, C. W. and Cerny, J. C.: Congenital absence of abdominal muscles: Report of 6 cases. J. Urol. 98:252-259, 1967.
39. Boyarsky, S.: *The Neurogenic Bladder.* Baltimore, Williams and Wilkins, 1967.
40. Boyce, W. H., Lathem, E. J. and Hunt, L. D.: Research related to an artificial electrical stimulator for the paralyzed human bladder. J. Urol. 91:41-51, 1964.
41. Bozler, E.: Action potentials and conduction of excitation in muscle. Biol. Sympos. 3:95-110, 1941.
42. Bozler, E.: The activity of the pacemaker previous to the discharge of a muscular impulse. Amer. J. Physiol. 136:543-552, 1942.
43. Bozler, E.: Conduction, automaticity and tonus of visceral muscles. Experientia 4:213-218, 1948.

44. Bracci, U.: Su le stenosi disontogenetiche dell'uretra maschile con particolare riguardo a quelle valvolari della porzione prostatica. Policlinico (Chir.) 45:554-576, 1938.
45. Bradley, W., Chou, S., Markland, C. and Swaiman, K.: Biochemical assay techniques for estimation of bladder fibrosis. Invest. Urol. 3:59-64, 1965.
46. Bradley, W. F. and Teague, C. T.: Innervation of the vesical detrusor muscle by the ganglia of the pelvic plexus. Invest. Urol. 6:251-266, 1968.
47. Bradley, W. F. and Teague, C. T.: Hypogastric and pelvic nerve activity during the micturition reflex. J. Urol. 102:438-440, 1969.
48. Braithwaite, J. L.: The arterial supply of the male urinary bladder. Brit. J. Urol. 24:64-71, 1952.
49. Bro-Rasmussen, F., Halborg Sorenson, A., Bredahl, E. and Kelstrup, A.: The structure and function of the urinary bladder. Urol. Int. 19:280-295, 1965.
50. Brosig, W.: Experimentelle Untersuchungen über den Blasentonus. Z. Urol. 46:456-466, 1953.
51. Bruézière, J. and Firmin, F.: Maladie du col vésical chez l'enfant. Etude clinique, diagnostique, thérapeutique. Ann. d'Urol. 4:169-186, 1970.
52. Bruton, O. C.: Agenesis of abdominal musculature associated with genito-urinary and gastrointestinal tract anomalies. J. Urol. 66:607-611, 1951.
53. Bryndorf, J. and Sandal, E.: The hydrodynamics of micturition. Danish Med. Bull. 7:65-71, 1960.
54. Bugbee, H. G. and Wollstein, M.: Retention of urine due to congenital hypertrophy of the verumontanum. J. Urol. 10:477-490, 1923.
55. Bugbee, H. G. and Wollstein, M.: Surgical pathology of the urinary tract in infants. J.A.M.A. 83:1887-1894, 1924.
56. Bulbring, E. J.: Correlation between membrane potential, spike discharge and tension in smooth muscle. J. Physiol. 128:200-221, 1955.
57. Bulloch, R. T., Davis, J. L. and Hara, M.: Dystrophia myotonia with heart block: A light and electron microscopy study. Arch. Path. 84:130-140, 1967.
58. Bulmer, D.: Observations on the lower end of the vagina in the sheep. J. Anat. 86:233-245, 1952.
59. Bulmer, D.: The early stages of vaginal development in the sheep. J. Anat. 90:123-134, 1956.
60. Bulmer, D.: The development of the human vagina. J. Anat. 91:490-509, 1957.
61. Bumpus, H. C., Jr.: Urinary reflux. J. Urol. 12:341-346, 1924.
62. Bunge, R. G.: Delayed cystograms in children. J. Urol. 70:729-732, 1953.
63. Bunting, C. H.: Chronic fibrous myocarditis in progressive muscular dystrophy. Amer. J. Med. Sci. 135:244-251, 1908.
64. Burkholder, G. V. and Harper, R. C.: Personal communication, 1970.
65. Burns, E. and Harvard, B. M.: Common congenital lesions of the urinary tract. J.A.M.A. 146:419-423, 1951.
66. Burns, E.: The modified retropubic operation for bladder neck obstruction in children. Urol. Survey 2:1, 1952.
67. Burns, E., Pratt, A. M. and Hendon, R. G.: Management of bladder neck obstruction in children. J.A.M.A. 157:570-574, 1955.
68. Burns, E., Ray, E. H. and Morgan, J. W.: Bladder neck obstruction and associated lesions in children. J. Urol. 77:733-740, 1957.
69. Burnstock, G. and Prosser, C. L.: Conduction in smooth muscles; comparative electrical properties. Amer. J. Physiol. 199:553-559, 1960.
70. Burnstock, G., Holman, M. E. and Prosser, C. L.: Electrophysiology of smooth muscle. Physiol. Rev. 43:482-527, 1963.
71. Burnstock, G. and Holman, M. E.: Effect of drugs on smooth muscle. Ann. Rev. Pharmacol. 6:129-156, 1966.
72. Burrows, E. H.: *Urethral Lesions in Infancy and Childhood*. Springfield, Charles C Thomas, 1965.

73. Caesar, R., Edwards, G. A. and Ruska, H.: Architecture and nerve supply of mammalian smooth muscle tissue. J. Biophys. Biochem. Cytol. 3:867-877, 1957.
74. Campbell, M. F.: Submucous fibrosis of the bladder outlet in infancy and childhood. J.A.M.A. 94:1373-1378, 1930.
75. Campbell, M. F.: Posterior urethral valve obstruction in infancy and in childhood: Study of eighteen cases. J.A.M.A. 96:592-597, 1931.
76. Campbell, M. F.: *Clinical Pediatric Urology*. Philadelphia, W. B. Saunders, 1951.
77. Campbell, M. F.: The diagnosis of early obstruction (contracture) of the bladder neck with particular consideration of trigonal changes. Southern Med. J. 57:76-78, 1964.
78. Cardus, D., Quesada, E. M. and Scott, F. B.: The use of the electromagnetic flowmeter for urine flow measurements. J. Appl. Physiol. 18:845-847, 1963.
79. Cardus, D., Quesada, E. M. and Scott, F. B.: Studies on the dynamics of the bladder. J. Urol. 90:425-433, 1963.
80. Caulk, J. R.: Fallacious orifice; contracture of the vesical neck. J. Urol. 14:293-299, 1925.
81. Caylor, H. D. and Walters, W.: Leiomyosarcoma of urinary bladder. J. Urol. 24:303-311, 1930.
82. Ceccarelli, F. E. and Beach, P. D.: Multiple urogenital anomalies; pronephric, mesonephric, and metanephric kidney elements with persistent müllerian duct in an adult male. J. Urol. 85:31-41, 1961.
83. Cendron, J. and Valayer, J.: Les vessies neurologiques chez l'enfant. Rev. Pediat. 6:425-432, 1968.
84. Chang, C. Y.: Anterior urethral valves: A case report. J. Urol. 100:29-31, 1968.
85. Chatelain, C., Mathieu, F. and Küss, R.: Maladie du col vésicale. Rev. Prat. 17:885-909, 1967.
86. Chauvin, H. F.: A propos de 10 cas de maladies du col chez l'enfant. J. Urol. Nephrol. 64:483-485, 1958.
87. Chetwood, C. H.: Prostatism without enlargement of the prostate. Ann. Surg. 41:497-506, 1905.
88. Chopra, H. C.: Investigations of the fine structure of smooth muscle fibers of prostate gland. Cellule 65:213-216, 1965.
89. Chwalla, R.: Case of amyloidosis at bladder neck resembling tumor. Urol. Cutan. Rev. 36:381-384, 1932.
90. Chwalla, R.: Die starre des innern Blasenschliessmuskels. Bericht über 30 operierte. Fälle and über die Dauerresultate der transvesikalen Keilexcision aus dem sphincter internus. Beitr. Klin. Chir. 147:579-619, 1929.
91. Clegg, E. J.: The musculature of the human prostatic urethra. J. Anat. 91:345-351, 1957.
92. Cobb, B. G., Wolf, J. A., Jr. and Ansell, J. S.: Congenital stricture of the proximal urethral bulb. J. Urol. 99:629-631, 1968.
93. Cockett, A. T. K.: The urological problems in space medicine. J. Urol. 92:564-567, 1964.
94. Colabawalla, B. N.: Anterior urethral valve: A case report. J. Urol. 94:58-60, 1965.
95. Collings, C. W.: Fibrous obstruction of the vesical outlet. New Eng. J. Med. 203:107-114, 1930.
96. Comar, A. E.: The practical management of the patient with spinal cord injury. Brit. J. Urol. 31:1-46, 1959.
97. Conger, K. B. and Toub, L.: Obstruction of the bladder neck in the male infant and child: Present concepts of diagnostic methods of management and a report of 14 cases. J. Pediat. 57:855-875, 1960.
98. Connor, R. C. R. and Adams, J. H.: Importance of cardiomyopathy and cerebral ischaemia in the diagnosis of fatal coma in pregnancy. J. Clin. Path. 19:244-249, 1966.

99. Conway, C. J. and Bradley, W. E.: Measurement of spread of excitation of the urinary detrusor muscle during reflex induction. J. Urol. 101:533-538, 1969.
100. Cook, F. E. and Shaw, J. L.: Cystic anomalies of the ducts of Cowper's glands. J. Urol. 85:659-664, 1961.
100a. Corrin, B., Mayor, D. and Moore T.: The pathology of bladder neck obstruction in the female patient. J. Urol. 90:434-439, 1963.
101. Cowper, W.: An account of two glands and their excretory ducts lately discovered in human bodies. Philos. Trans. Brit. Roy. Soc. 258:364, 1699.
102. Csapó, A.: Actomyosin of the uterus. Amer. J. Physiol. 160:46-52, 1950.
103. Csapó, A.: Molecular structure in function of smooth muscle. In *Muscle*, Vol. I (Bourne, G. H., Ed.). New York, Academic Press, 1960.
104. Cukier, J., Maury, M., Audic, B. and Baccialone, L.: La miction après les sections médullaires complètes. J. Urol. Nephrol. 78:515-549, 1964.
105. Culp, D. A. and Flocks, R. H.: Congenital absence of abdominal musculature; report of 2 cases. Iowa State Med. Soc. 44:155-159, 1954.
106. Cussen, L. J.: The structure of the normal human ureter in infancy and childhood. Invest. Urol. 5:179-194, 1967.
107. Daniel, J., Stewart, A. M. and Blair, D. W.: Congenital anterior urethral valve—Diagnosis and treatment. Brit. J. Urol. 40:589-591, 1968.
107a. Davies, J. and Kusama, H.: Developmental aspects of the human cervix. Ann. N. Y. Acad. Sci. 97:534-550, 1962.
108. Davidsohn, I. and Newberger, C.: Congenital valves of the posterior urethra in twins. Arch. Path. 16:57-62, 1933.
109. Deakin, R.: Congenital bladder neck obstruction in children. J. Urol. 78:384-392, 1957.
110. Dell'Adami, G.: *Le Alterazzioni Ostruttive Delle Vie Urinarie Escretici Nell'Infanzia*. Padova, Piccin, 1959.
111. DeLuca, F. G., Swenson, O., Fisher, J. H. and Loutfi, A. H.: The dysfunctional "lazy" bladder syndrome in children. Arch. Dis. Child. 37:117-121, 1962.
112. Deniz, E., Shimkus, G. J. and Weller, R.: Pelvic neurofibromatosis: Localized von Recklinghausen's disease of the bladder. J. Urol. 96:906-909, 1966.
113. Denny-Brown, D. and Robertson, E. G.: On the physiology of micturition. Brain 56:149-190, 1933.
114. Denny-Brown, D. E.: Nervous disturbances of the vesical sphincter. New Eng. J. Med. 215:647-650, 1936.
115. DeWeerd, J. H.: Heineke-Mikulicz principle applied to retropubic revision of the vesical neck. J. Urol. 95:368-373, 1966.
116. Dewey, M. M. and Barr, L. A.: A study of the structure and distribution of the nexus. J. Cell. Biol. 23:553-585, 1964.
117. Disse, J.: Harnorgane. In *Bardeleben's Handbuch der Anatomie des Menschen*, Vol. 7. Jena, Fischer, 1904.
118. Dogiel, A. S.: Über den bau der ganglien in den geflechten des darmes und der gallenblase des menschen und der säugetier. Z. Anat. Entwickl. 130-158, 1899.
119. Donahue, J. P. and Leadbetter, Guy W., Jr.: An evaluation of voiding cystometry as a diagnostic test for bladder outlet obstruction. J. Urol. 92:464-472, 1964.
120. Downs, R. A.: Congenital polyps of the prostatic urethra—A review of the literature and report of two cases. Brit. J. Urol. 42:76-85, 1970.
121. Drake, W. M., Jr.: The uroflometer: an aid to the study of the lower urinary tract. J. Urol. 59:650-658, 1948.
122. Dyson, B. C. and Decker, J. P.: Endocardial fibroelastosis in the adult. Arch. Path. 66:190-203, 1958.
123. Eagle J. F., Jr. and Barrett, G. S.: Congenital deficiency of abdominal musculature with associated genito-urinary abnormalities: A syndrome. Report of nine cases. Pediatrics 6:721-736, 1950.
124. Eberth, C. J.: Die männlichen Geschlechtsorgane. In *Bardeleben's Handbuch der Anatomie des Meschen*. Vol. 7. Jena, Fischer, 1904.

125. Eckstein, H. B.: Urinary control in children with myelomeningocele. Brit. J. Urol. 41:191-195, 1968.
126. Edling. N. P. G.: Urethrocystography in the male with special regard to micturition. Acta Radiol. Suppl. 58, 1945.
127. Edling, N. P. G.: Radiological aspects of the utriculus prostaticus during urethrocystography. Acta Radiol. 32:28-32, 1949.
128. Edling, N. P. G.: The radiologic appearances of diverticula of the male cavernous urethra. Acta Radiol. 40:1-8, 1953.
129. Edwards, D.: Cinéradiography of the congenital neurogenic bladder. Proc. Roy. Soc. Med. 49:898-899, 1956.
130. Eisenstaedt, J. S.: Primary congenital megaloureters. Arch. Surg. 13:64-74, 1926.
131. El-Badawi, A. and Schenk, E. A.: Dual innervation of the mammalian bladder. A histochemical study of the distribution of cholinergic and adrenergic nerves. Amer. J. Anat. 119:405-428, 1966.
132. Elbogen, A.: Zur Kentniss der Cystenbildung aus den Ausführungsgängen der Cowper schen Drüsen. Z. Kinderheilk. 7:221-224, 1886.
133. Elliot, J. S.: Postoperative urinary incontinence: A revised concept of the external sphincter. J. Urol. 71:49-57, 1954.
134. Elliot, T. R.: The innervation of the bladder and urethra. J. Physiol. 35:367-445, 1907.
135. Emmet. J. L.: Obstruction of the vesical neck of a male infant produced by hypertrophy of the verumontanum: Report of a case. Mayo Clin. Proc. June 5, 1940.
136. Emmet, J. L., Daut, R. V. and Dunn, J. H.: Role of the external urethral sphincter in the normal bladder and cord bladder. J. Urol. 59:439-454, 1948.
137. Emmet, J. L. and Helmholz, H. F.: Transurethral resection of the vesical neck in infants and children. J. Urol. 60:463-478, 1948.
138. Emmet, J. L. and Simon, H. B.: Transurethral resection in infants and children for congenital obstruction of the vesical neck and myelodysplasia. J. Urol. 76:595-608, 1956.
139. Englisch. J.: Cited by Neustein, D. H. and Schutte, H.: Müllerian duct cyst. Brit. J. Urol. 40:72-77, 1968.
140. Englisch, J.: Uber retentioncysten der ausfürhengängen bei der Cowperischen drüsen. Tagebl. Deutsch. Naturforsch. Aerst. 54:148, 1881.
141. Enhörning, G.: Simultaneous recording of intravesical and intraurethral pressure. Acta Chir. Scand. Suppl. 276, 1961.
142. Ericsson, N. O.: Ectopic ureterocele in infants and children. Acta Chir. Scand. Suppl. 197, 1954.
143. Ericsson, N. O.: Congenital urethral obstruction. Acta Urol. Belg. 30:316-325, 1962.
144. Evans, C. L.: The physiology of plain muscle. Physiol. Rev. 6:358-398, 1926.
145. Evans, J. P.: Observations on the nerves of supply to the bladder and urethra of the cat with a study of their action potentials. J. Physiol. 86:396-414, 1936.
146. Eyrick, T. B., Many, M. and Wise, H. M., Jr.: Analysis of urethral resistance: A clinically applicable method for evaluation of urethral dynamics. Invest. Urol. 6:443-465, 1969.
147. Felix, W.: Development of the urogenital organs. In *Human Embryology*, 2nd ed. (Keibel-Mall, Eds.). Philadelphia, J. B. Lippincott, 1912.
148. Finkle, A. L., McPhee, V. G. and van der Reis, L.: Congenital bladder neck contracture in male siblings. Calif. Med. 85:260-264, 1956.
149. Firestone, A.: The neglected bulbo-urethral glands of Cowper. Urol. Cutan. Rev. 42:231-232, 1938.
150. Fisher, O. D. and Forsythe, W. I.: Micturating cysto-urethrography in investigation of enuresis. Arch. Dis. Child. 29:460-471, 1954.
151. Flanagan, M. J., Kiefer, J. H. and McDonald, J. H.: Pedunculated solid polyp of posterior urethra. J. Urol. 90:200-202, 1963.

152. Fletcher, W. M. A.: Congenital absence of abdominal wall. Med. J. Aust. 1:435-436, 1928.
153. Flocks, R. H.: Lower urinary tract obstruction in infants and children. Pediat. Clin. N. Amer. 2:755-770, 1955.
154. Flocks, R. H., Prendergast, L. J., Marberger, H. and Culp, D.: Newer methods for treatment of urethral stricture. Arch. Surg. 71:109-114, 1955.
155. Forsberg, J. G.: Mitotic rate and autoradiographic studies on the derivation and differentiation of the epithelium of the mouse vaginal anlage. Acta Anat. 62:266-282, 1965.
156. Frankel, H. H., Benick, S., Patek, P. R., Edmondson, H. A., Peters, R. L. and Paule, W. J.: Elastic membranes of the developing human aorta. Arch. Path. 76:474-483, 1963.
157. Franksson, C. and Petersén, I.: Electromyographic recording from the normal urinary bladder, internal urethral sphincter and ureter. Acta Physiol. Scand. 29 (Suppl. 106):150-156, 1953.
158. Franksson, C. and Petersén. I.: Electromyographic investigation of disturbances in the striated muscle of the urethral sphincter. Brit. J. Urol. 27:154-161, 1955.
159. Frazer, J. E.: The terminal part of the wolffian duct. J. Anat. 69:455-468, 1935.
160. Fredericks, C. M., Anderson, G. F., Rasmussen, E. A. and Pierce, J. M.: Electrophysiology of the canine urinary bladder. Invest. Urol. 7:33-40, 1969.
161. Friedel, A.: Die entleerung der harnblase nach Heiss. Med. Klin. 25:1396, 1929.
162. Frölich, F.: *Der Mangel der Muskeln, Insbesondere der Seitenbauchmuskeln.* Wurzburg, C. A. Zurn, 1939.
163. Fuchs, N.: Zwei fälle von Kongenitaler hydronephrose. Cited by Knox, J. H. and Sprunt, T. P.: Amer. J. Dis. Child. 4:137-147, 1912.
164. Fuller, E.: Cited by Borm, D. and Clausen, E.: Die Blasensphinktersklerose. Bruns Beitr. Klin. Chir. 4:447-468, 1963.
165. Gansler, H.: Beitrag zur Struktur der glatten muskelzelle. Proc. Stockholm Conf. 210-212, 1956.
166. Gansler, H.: Phase contrast and electron microscopic studies on morphology and function of smooth musculature. Z. Zellforsch. 52:60-91, 1960.
167. Garrett, R. A., Rhamy, R. K. and Newman, D.: Management of nonobstructive vesicoureteral reflux. J. Urol. 90:167-172, 1963.
168. Giertz, G. and Lindblom K.: Urethrocystographic studies of nervous disturbances of the urinary bladder and the urethra: A preliminary report. Acta Radiol. 36:205-216, 1951.
169. Gil Vernet, S.: Union ureterotrigonal esfinter ureteral prevesical. Arch. Esp. Urol. 23:1-64, 1970.
170. Gil Vernet, S.: *Patologia Urogenital*, Tomo I. Barcelona, Miguel Servet, 1944.
171. Gil Vervet, S.: *Patologia Urogenital*, Tomo II. Madrid, Paz. Montalvo, 1953.
172. Gil Vernet, S.: *Patologia Urogenital*, Tomo II. Madrid, Paz. Montalvo, 1955.
173. Gil Vernet, S.: Physiologie der Miktion. Z. Urol. 53:181-202, 1960.
174. Gil Vernet, S.: L'innervation somatique et végétative des organes genitourinaires. Acta Urol. Belg. 32:265-293, 1964.
175. Gil Vernet, S.: Maladie du col vésical ou prostatisme sans hypértrophie de la prostate. Urol. Int. 18:216-226, 1964.
176. Gil Vernet, S.: *Morphology and Function of Vesico-prostato-urethral Musculature* Treviso, Edizioni Canova, 1968.
177. Gireaux, B.: Personal communication (unpublished thesis).
178. Gleason, D. M. and Lattimer, J. K.: The pressure flow study: A method for measuring bladder neck resistance. J. Urol. 87:844-852, 1962.
179. Gleason, D. M. and Lattimer, J. K.: A miniature radio transmitter which is inserted into the bladder and records voiding pressures. J. Urol. 87:507-509, 1962.
180. Gleason, D. M. and Lattimer, J. K.: The interpretation of voiding pressure. J. Urol. 91:156-160, 1964.

181. Gleason, D. M., Lattimer, J. K. and Bauxbaum, C.: Bladder pressure telemetry. J. Urol. 94:252-256, 1965.
182. Gleason, D. M., Bottaccini, M. R., Perling, D. and Lattimer, J. K.: A challenge to current urodynamic thought. J. Urol. 97:935-940, 1967.
183. Gleason, D. M. and Bottaccini, M. R.: The vital role of the distal urethral segment in the control of urinary flow rate. J. Urol. 100:167-170, 1968.
184. Gleason, D. M., Bottaccini, M. R. and Lattimer, J. K.: Some correlations between the hydrodynamic and clinical findings in the urinary tract. J. Urol. 100:783-786, 1968.
185. Glenn, J. F. and Montgomery, W. G.: A clinical classification of bladder outlet obstruction, J. Urol. 91:232-240, 1964.
186. Glenn, J. F. and Anderson, E. E.: Distal tunnel ureteral reimplantation. J. Urol. 97:623-626, 1967.
187. Glenn, J. F. and Boyce, W. H.: *Urologic Surgery.* New York, Hoeber, 1969.
188. Glingar, A.: *Wiener Beiträge zur Urologie.* Vienna, Wilhelm Mandrich, 1947.
189. Gomez-Oliveros, L.: Über den bau der blasenhalsmuskulatur und der harnröhrensphinkteren beim Mann. Med. Welt 20:1201-1205, 1969.
190. Grasset, D.: *La Cysto-sphinctérométrie. Exploration Dynamique de l'Appareil Vesico-sphinctérien.* Paris, Masson et Cie., 1961.
191. Grasset, D.: Les obstructions du bas appareil urinaire chez l'enfant. In *Rapport a l'Association Francaise d'Urologie,* 64e Session. Paris, Masson et Cie., 1970.
192. Greene, L. F., Emmett, J. L., Culp, O. S. and Kennedy, R. L. J.: Congenital absence of abdominal muscles with urologic complications: In *Collected Papers of the Mayo Clinic and the Mayo Foundation.* Philadelphia, W. B. Saunders, 1953.
193. Griesback, W. A., Waterhouse, R. K. and Mellins, H. Z.: Voiding cystourethrography in the diagnosis of congenital posterior urethral valves. Amer. J. Roentgen. 82:521-529, 1959.
194. Gross, R. E., Randolph, J. and Wise, H. M., Jr.: Surgical correction of bladder neck obstruction in children. New Eng. J. Med. 268:5-14, 1963.
195. Gruenwald, P.: The relation of the growing müllerian duct to the wolffian duct and its importance for the genesis of malformations. Anat. Rec. 81:1-20, 1941.
196. Gute, D. B., Chute, R. and Baron, J. A.: Bladder neck revision for obstruction in men: A clinical study reporting normal ejaculation post-operatively. J. Urol. 99:744-749, 1968.
197. Guthrie, G. J.: *On the Anatomy and Disease of the Neck of the Bladder and Urethra.* London, Burgess and Hill, 1834.
198. Guyon, J. C. F.: *Lecons Cliniques sur les Affections Chirurgicales de la Vessie et de la Prostate.* Paris, F. P. Guiard, 1888.
199. Gyllensten, L.: Contributions to the embryology of the urinary bladder. Acta Anat. 7:305-344, 1949.
200. Habib, H. N.: Neural trigger points for evacuation of neurogenic bladder by electro-stimulation. Surg. Forum 14:489-492, 1963.
201. Haines, R. W.: The striped compressor of the prostatic urethra. Brit. J. Urol. 61:481-493, 1969.
202. Hald, T., Freed, P. S. and Kantrowitz, A.: Urinary bladder: Mode of excitation during stimulation. Invest. Urol. 4:239-246, 1966.
203. Hall, D. A., Reed, R. and Tunbridge, R. E.: Electron microscope studies of elastic tissue. Exp. Cell. Res. 8:35-48, 1955.
204. Hall, D. A.: Collagen and elastin: The effect of age on their relationship. Gerontologia 1:347-363, 1957.
205. Hall, D. A.: *Elastolysis and Aging.* Springfield, Charles C Thomas, 1964.
206. Hamilton, W. J., Boyd, J. D. and Mossman, H. W. *Human Embryology.* Cambridge, W. Heffer and Sons, Ltd., 1959.
207. Hand, J. R. and Sullivan, A. W.: Retropubic prostatectomy: Analysis of 100 cases. J.A.M.A. 145:1313-1321, 1951.
208. Hanson, J. and Huxley, H. E.: Structural basis of the cross-striations in muscle. Nature 172:530-532, 1953.

209. Hanson, J. and Lowy, J.: Structure of muscle fibers in translucent part of adductor of the oyster Crassotrea angulata. Proc. Roy. Soc. 154:173-196, 1961.
210. Hanson, J. and Lowy, J.: The structure of F- actin and of actin filaments isolated from smooth muscle. J. Molec. Biol. 6:46-60, 1963.
211. Hanson, J. and Lowy, J.: The structure of actin filaments and the origin of the axial periodicity in the I-substance of vertebrate striated muscle. Proc. Roy. Soc. 160:449-460, 1964.
212. Hanten, J. S., Galuszka, A. A. and Rotner, M.: Vesical neck obstruction in children. J. Urol. 82:218-223, 1959.
213. Harman, J. W., O'Hegarty, M. T. and Byrnes, C. K.: The ultrastructure of human smooth muscle. 1. Studies of cell surface and connections in normal and achalasia esophageal smooth muscle. Exp. Molec. Path. 1:204-228, 1962.
214. Harrison, F. G.: Urinary obstruction in children inducing renal hyperparathyroidism. J. Urol. 48:44-57, 1942.
215. Harrow, R., Sloane, J. A. and Wittus, W. S.: Congenital dilatation of the female urethra. J. Urol. 95:58-62, 1966.
216. Harrow, B. R.: The myth of the megacystis syndrome. J. Urol. 98:205, 1967.
217. Hasen, H. B. and Song, Y. S.: Congenital valvular obstruction of the posterior urethra in two brothers. J. Pediat. 47:207-215, 1955.
218. Hayek, H.: Zur anatomie des sphincter urethrae. Z. Anat. Entwick. 123:121-125, 1962.
219. Headstream, J. W.: Obstruction of the bladder neck in children. Postgrad. Med. J.: 28:457-469, 1960.
220. Heiss, R.: Über den sphincter vesicae. Virchow Arch. Path. Anat. 5-6:367-383, 1915.
221. Henle, J.: *Handbuch der Systematischen Anatomie des Menschen,* Vol. 2. Braunschweig, Friedrich Vieweg, 1866.
222. Henley, W. L. and Hyman, A.: Absent abdominal musculature, genitourinary anomalies, and deficiency in pelvic autonomic nervous system. Amer. J. Dis. Child. 86:795-798, 1953.
223. Hennig, von O.: Neuere anatomische und physiologische Erkenntnisse über Prostata und Blasenauslass und Ihrer Bedeutung für operative Eingriffe. Z. Urol. 47:457-477, 1954.
224. Hinman, F.: *The Principles and Practice of Urology.* Philadelphia, W. B. Saunders, 1935.
225. Hinman, F. J., Jr. and Miller, E. R.: Mural tension in vesical disorders and ureteral reflux. J. Urol. 91:33-40, 1964.
226. Hodgkinson, C. P.: Direct urethrocystometry. Amer. J. Obstet. Gynec. 79:648-664, 1960.
227. Hofstein, J.: Absence congénitale des muscles abdominaux chez un nouveau-né, du sexe féminin. Gynec. Obstet. 22:23-28, 1930.
228. Holm, H. H.: Micro-manometer for the measurement of intravesical pressure. J. Urol. 86:280-285, 1962.
229. Holm, H. H.: The hydrodynamics of micturition. Acta Radiol., Suppl. 231, 1964.
230. Hope, J. W., Jameson, P. J. and Michie, A. J.: Voiding urethrography: An integral part of intravenous urography. J. Pediat. 56:768-773, 1960.
231. Hope, J. W., Jameson, P. J. and Michie, A. J.: Diagnosis of anterior urethral valve by voiding urethrography: Report of two cases. Radiology, 74:798-801, 1960.
232. Hosli, O. P.: Die fibro-elastose des blasenhals beim männlichen säugling ("Marionische Krankheit"). Urol. Int. 11:240-252, 1961.
233. Howard, F. S.: Hypospadias with enlargement of the prostatic utricle. Surg. Gynec. Obstet. 86:307:316, 1948.
234. Howard. P. J.: Congenital absence of the abdominal muscles and genito-urinary malformation: Report of 2 cases. Amer. J. Dis. Child. 60:669-676, 1940.
235. Howard, T. L. and Buchtel, H. A.: Resection of vesical neck in children: Indications and results. J.A.M.A. 146:1202-1206, 1951.

236. Howerton, L. and Lich, R., Jr.: The cause and correction of ureteral reflux. J. Urol. 89:673-675, 1963.
237. Huffman, G. C. and Keitzer, W.: Urodynamics of the lower urinary tract. Invest. Urol. 3:1-9, 1965.
238. Hunter, DeW. T., Jr.: A new concept of the urinary bladder musculature. J. Urol. 71:695-704, 1954.
239. Hutch, J. A.: Vesico-ureteral reflux in the paraplegic: Cause and correction. J. Urol. 68:457-467, 1952.
240. Hutch, J. A.: *The Ureterovesical Junction*. Berkeley, Univ. of California Press, 1958.
241. Hutch, J. A.: Theory of maturation of the intravesical ureter. J. Urol. 86:534-538, 1961.
242. Hutch, J. A., Miller, E. R. and Hinman, F., Jr.: Perpetuation of infection in obstructed urinary tracts by vesico-ureteral reflux. J. Urol. 90:88-91, 1963.
243. Hutch, J. A.: A new theory of the anatomy of the internal sphincter and the physiology of micturition. Invest. Urol. 3:36-58, 1965.
244. Hutch, J. A. and Shopfner, C. E.: A new theory of the anatomy of the internal urinary sphincter and the physiology of micturition VI. The base plate and enuresis. J. Urol. 99:174-177, 1968.
245. Hutch, J. A. and Shopfner, C. E.: The lateral cystogram as an aid to urologic diagnosis. J. Urol. 99:292-296, 1968.
246. Hutch, J. A. and Elliott, H. W.: Electromyographic study of electrical activity in the para-urethral muscles prior to and during voiding. J. Urol. 99:759-765, 1968.
247. Hutch, J. A.: The internal sphincter: A double loop system. Trans. Amer. Assoc. Genitourin. Surg. 62:30-38, 1970.
248. Huvos, A. G. and Pruzanski, W.: Smooth muscle involvement in primary muscle disease. III. Myasthenia gravis. Arch. Path. 84:280-285, 1967.
249. Huvos, A. G. and Pruzanski, W.: Smooth muscle involvement in primary muscle disease: II. Progressive muscular dystrophy. Arch. Path. 83:234-240, 1967.
250. Huxley, H. and Hanson, J.: Changes in the cross-striations of muscle during contraction and stretch and their structural interpretation. Nature 173:973-976, 1954.
251. Huxley, H. E.: Personal communication, 1961.
252. Ikeda, K. and Stoesser, A. V.: Congenital defect in musculature of abdominal wall. Amer. J. Dis. Child. 33:286-293, 1927.
253. Irisawa, H. and Kobayashi, M.: Effects of repetitive stimuli and temperature on ureter action potentials. Jap. J. Physiol. 13:421-430, 1963.
254. Johnson, F. P.: Diverticula and cysts of the glands of Cowper. J. Urol. 10:295-302, 1923.
255. Johnson, S. H., III, and Price, W. C.: Hypertrophy of the colliculus seminalis in childhood. Amer. J. Dis. Child. 78:892-898, 1950.
256. Johnston, J. H.: Posterior urethral valves: Operative technique with electric auriscope. J. Pediat. Surg. 1:583-584, 1966.
257. Jones, B. W. and Headstream. J. W.: Vesicoureteral reflux in children. J. Urol. 80:114-116, 1958.
258. Jones, H. W., Jr. and Scott, W. W.: *Hermaphroditism, Genital Anomalies and Related Endocrine Disorders*. Baltimore, Williams and Wilkins, 1958.
259. Kalischer, O.: *Die Urogenital Musculatur des Dammes, mit Besonderer Berücksichtigung des Harnblasenverschlusses*. Berlin, S. Karger, 1900.
260. Kantrowitz, A.: Development of an implantable, externally controlled stimulator for the treatment of chronic cord bladder in paraplegic patients; report of three cases. Arch. Phys. Med. 46:76-78, 1965.
261. Kantrowitz, A. and Schamaun, M.: Bladder evacuation in paraplegic dogs by direct electric stimulation. J.A.M.A. 187:595-597, 1964.
262. Kaufman, C.: *Verletzungen und Krankheiten der Maennlichen Harnroehre und des Penis*. Stuttgart, Enke, 1886.

263. Kaufman, J. J.: A new uroflometer. A simple automatic device for measuring voiding velocity. J. Urol. 78:97-102, 1957.
264. Karlson, S.: Experimental studies on the functioning of the female urinary bladder and urethra. Acta Obstet. Gynec. Scand. 32:285-307, 1953.
265. Keech, M. K. and Wood, M. J.: Further observations on the transformation of collagen fibrils into "elastin": An electronmicroscopic study. J. Path. Bact. 71:477-493, 1956.
266. Keitzer, W. A. and Benavent, C.: Bladder neck obstruction in children. J. Urol. 89:384-388, 1963.
267. Keitzer, W. A. and Huffman, G. C.: The voiding audiograph: A new voiding test. J. Urol. 96:404-410, 1966.
268. Kerr, H. D. and Gillis, C. L.: *The Urinary Tract*. Chicago, Year Book Medical Publishers, 1944.
269. King, L. R.: Idiopathic dilatation of posterior urethra in boys without bladder outlet obstruction. J. Urol. 102:783-787, 1969.
270. King, L. R., Mellins, H. Z. and Scott, W. W.: Radiographic evaluation of the bladder neck in childhood. J. Urol. 91:52-57, 1964.
271. King, L. R., Mellins, H. Z. and White, H.: Measurement of intravesical pressure during voiding. Invest. Urol. 2:303-322, 1965.
272. Kjellberg, S. R., Ericsson, H. O. and Rudhe, U.: *The Lower Urinary Tract in Childhood: Some Correlated Clinical and Roentgenologic Observations*. Chicago, Year Book Medical Publishers, 1957.
273. Kleeman, F. J.: The physiology of the internal urinary sphincter. J. Urol. 104:549-554, 1970.
274. Knox, J. H., Jr. and Sprunt, T. P.: Congenital obstruction of the posterior urethra: A report of a case in a boy aged five years. Amer. J. Dis. Child. 4:137-147, 1912.
275. Kobayashi, M.: Conduction velocity in various regions of the ureter. Tohoku J. Exp. Med. 83:220-224, 1964.
276. Kobayashi, M. and Irisawa, H.: Effect of sodium deficiency on the action potential of the smooth muscle of ureter. Amer. J. Physiol. 206:205-210, 1964.
277. Kobayashi, M.: Effects of Na and Ca on the generation and conduction of excitation in the ureter. Amer. J. Physiol. 208:715-719, 1965.
278. Kock, N. G. and Pompeius, R.: Studies on the rhythmic activity of the human bladder. Invest. Urol. 1:253-261, 1963.
279. Koff, A.: Development of the vagina in the human foetus. Contrib. Embryol. Carnegie Inst., 24:59-91, 1933.
280. Kohlrausch, O.: *Zur Anatomie und Physiologie der Beckenorgane*. Leipzig, Hirzel, 1854.
281. Krahn, H. P. and Morales, P. A.: The effect of pudendal nerve anesthesia on urinary continence after prostatectomy. J. Urol. 94:282-285, 1965.
282. Kretschmer, H. L. and Greer, J. R.: Insufficiency at the ureterovesical junction. Surg. Gynec. Obstet. 21:228-231, 1915.
283. Kretschmer, H. L. and Doerhing, P.: Leiomyosarcoma of urinary bladder. Arch. Surg. 38:274-286, 1939.
284. Kreutzmann, H. A. R.: Renal back pressure. Conclusive evidence as to its cause in obstructive lesions of the bladder neck and urethra. J.A.M.A. 92:213-216, 1929.
285. Krzeski, T.: Bladder neck obstruction in children. Acta Urol. Belg. 30:301-315, 1962.
286. Kultschizny, N.: Ueber die Art. der Verbindung der glatten Muskelfasern miteinander. Biol. Zentralbl. 7:572-574, 1887.
287. Kuntz, A. and Moseley, R. L.: An experimental analysis of the pelvic autonomic ganglia in the cat. J. Comp. Neurol. 64:63-75, 1936.
288. Kuntz, A. and Succomano, G.: The sympathetic innervation of the detrusor muscle. J. Urol. 51:535-542, 1944.
289. Langer, C. R. Von Edenberg: Cited by Pagano, F.: Le valvole congenite dell'uretra. Urologia, 16:72, 1965.

290. Länger-Toldt, D. T.: *Lehrbuch der Systematischen und Topographische Anatomie.* 3:Aufl. Hannover, 1893.
291. Langenbeck, Von, B. R. K.: Cited by Grasset, D.: Les obstructions du bas appareil urinaire chez l'enfant. In *Rapport a l'Association Francaise d'Urologie*, 64e Session. Paris, Masson et Cie., 1970.
292. Langworthy, O. R. and Murphy, E. L.: Nerve endings in the urinary bladder. J. Comp. Neurol. 71:487-505, 1939.
293. Langworthy, O. R., Kolb, L. C. and Lewis, L. G.: *Physiology of Micturition. Experimental and Clinical Studies with Suggestions as to Diagnosis and Treatment.* Baltimore, Williams and Wilkins, 1940.
294. Lansing, A. E., Rosenthal, T. B. and Dempsey, E. W.: The structure and chemical characterization of elastic fibers as revealed by elastase and by electron microscopy. Anat. Rec. 114:551-557, 1952.
295. Lapides, J.: Observations on normal and abnormal bladder physiology. J. Urol. 70:74-83, 1953.
296. Lapides, J., Sweet, R. B. and Lewis, L. W.: Role of striated muscle in urination. J. Urol. 77:247-250, 1957.
297. Lapides, J., Sweet, R. B. and Lewis, L. W.: Function of striated muscle in control of urination: II: Effect of complete skeletal muscle paralysis. Surg. Forum 6:313-315, 1955.
298. Lapides, J., Gray, H. O. and Rawling, J. C.: Function of striated muscles in control of urination. I: Effect of pudendal block. Surg. Forum 6:611-612, 1955.
299. Lapides, J.: Structure and function of the internal vesical sphincter, J. Urol. 80:341-353, 1958.
300. Lapides, J., Friend, C., Ajemian, E. and Reus, W.: A new test for neurogenic bladder. J. Urol. 88:245-247, 1962.
301. Lapides, J., Ajemian, E. P., Stewart, B. H., Breakey, B. A. and Lichtwardt, J. R.: Further observations on the kinetics of the urethrovesical sphincter. J. Urol. 84:86-94, 1960.
302. Lattimer, J. K.: Similar urogenital anomalies in identical twins. Amer. J. Dis. Child. 67:199-201, 1944.
303. Lattimer, J. K.: Congenital deficiency of the abdominal musculature and associated genito-urinary anomalies: A report of 22 cases. J. Urol. 79:343-352, 1958.
304. Leadbetter, G. W., Jr. and Leadbetter, W. F.: Diagnosis and treatment of congenital bladder-neck obstruction in children. New Eng. J. Med. 260:633-637, 1959.
305. Leadbetter, G. W., Jr. and Leadbetter, W. F.: Urethral strictures in male children. J. Urol. 87:409-415, 1962.
306. Leadbetter, G. W., Jr.: The etiology, symptoms and treatment of urethral strictures in male children. Pediatrics 31:80-86, 1963.
307. Leadbetter, G. W., Jr.: Urinary tract infection and obstruction in children. Clin. Pediat. 5:377-384, 1966.
308. Leadbetter, W. F.: Surgical management of simple reflux: Indications, objectives, technique, follow-up and results. In *Ureteral Reflux in Children* (Glenn, J. F., Ed.). Washington, National Academy of Sciences-National Research Council, 1966.
309. Learmonth, J. R.: A contribution to the neurophysiology of the urinary bladder in man. Brain 54:147-176, 1931.
310. Lebrèton, P.: Contribution à l'étude des glandes bulbo-uréthrales et leur maladies. Thèse de Paris 239, 1903-1904.
311. Legueu, F.: L'hypertrophie du col vésical. J. Urol. Nephrol. 24:534-539, 1927.
312. Le Gros-Clark, F.: Some remarks on the anatomy and physiology of the urinary bladder and sphincters of the rectum. J. Anat. Physiol. 17:442-459, 1883.
313. Legueu, F. and Dossot.: La dysectasie du col vésicale. Presse Med. 39:89-91, 1931.
314. Leibowitz, S. and Bodian, M.: A study of the vesical neck ganglia in children and the relationship to the megaureter-megacystis syndrome and Hirschsprung's disease. J. Clin. Path. 16:342-350, 1963.

315. Le Poutre, C.: Dilatation de l'arbre urinarie et reflux vesico-urétéral d'origine congénitale. J. Urol. Nephrol. 33:560-563, 1932.
316. Lich, R., Jr., Maurer, J. E. and Burdon, S.: Retropubic approach to vesical neck pathology in children. Brit. J. Urol. 22:21-25, 1950.
317. Lich, R., Jr. and Maurer, J. E.: Surgical relief of vesical neck obstruction in children. Southern Surg. 16:127-131, 1950.
318. Lich, R., Jr., Howerton, L. W. and Davis, L. A.: Vesicourethrography. J. Urol. 85:396-397, 1961.
319. Lich, R., Jr., Howerton, L. W., Jr., Goode, L. S. and Davis, L. A.: The uretero-vesical junction of the newborn. J. Urol. 92:435-438, 1964.
320. Lichtenstein, B. W.: Congenital absence of the abdominal musculature: Associated changes in the genito-urinary tract and in the spinal cord. Amer. J. Dis. Child. 58:339-348, 1939.
321. Lloyd-Davies, R. W., Clark, A. E., Prout, W. G., Shuttleworth, K. E. D. and Tighe, J. R.: The effects of stretching the rabbit bladder: Preliminary observations. Invest. Urol. 8:145-152, 1970.
322. Lowsley, O. S.: Congenital malformation of the posterior urethra. Ann. Surg. 60:733-741, 1914.
323. Lowsley, O. S. and Kirwin, T. J.: A clinical and pathological study of congenital obstruction of the urethra: Report of four cases. J. Urol. 31:497-516, 1934.
324. Lowsley, O. S. and Kirwin, T. J.: *Clinical Urology*, Vol. I. Baltimore, Williams and Wilkins, 1944.
325. Lowy, J., Paulson, F. R. and Vibert, P. J.: Myosin filaments in vertebrate smooth muscle. Nature 225:1053-1054, 1970.
326. Lyon, R. P. and Smith, D. R.: Distal urethral stenosis. J. Urol. 89:414-421, 1963.
327. Lyon, R. P. and Tanagho, E. A.: Distal urethral stenosis in little girls. J. Urol. 93:379-387, 1965.
328. Malin, J. M. and Boyarsky, S.: The effects of cholinergic and adrenergic drug stimulation of detrusor muscle. Invest. Urol. 8:286-291, 1970.
329. MacAlpine, J. B.: The musculature of the bladder neck of the male in health and disease. Proc. Roy. Soc. Med. 28:35-56, 1934.
330. Manley, C. B., Jr.: The striated muscle of the prostate. J. Urol. 95:234-240, 1966.
331. Marberger, H.: Stenosi congenita dell'uretera bulbare. Urologia, 9:1-9, 1959.
332. Marberger, H.: Blasenhalsplastik. Helv. Chir. Acta 28:768-771, 1960.
333. Marberger, H.: Die blasenhalsplastik nach Young. Langenbeck Arch. Klin. Chir. 298:638-642, 1961.
334. Marberger, H.: Bladder neck obstruction in childhood. Acta Urol. Belg. 31: 492-504, 1963.
335. Marberger, H.: Hydrodynamische probleme in der urologie von heute. Z. Urol. 58:871-876, 1965.
336. Marberger, H. and Madersbacher, H.: Beobachtungen über die Strömungsverhaltnisse am Blasenhals. Verh. Deutsch. Ges. Urol. 22:100-104, 1969.
337. Marion, G.: Surgery of neck of bladder. Brit. J. Urol. 5:351-356, 1933.
338. Marion, G.: In *Report Fifth Congress*, Société Internationale d'Urologie, 1933.
339. Marion, G.: *Traité d'Urologie*, 4ème ed. Paris, Masson et Cie, 1940.
340. Mark, J. S. T.: An electron microscope study of uterine smooth muscle. Anat. Rec. 125:473-493, 1956.
341. Markland, C., Chou, S., Bradley, W., Westgate, H. and Wolfson, J.: Some problems in the use of intermittent vesical electronic stimulation. Invest. Urol. 4:168-173, 1969.
342. Marshall, V. F.: Management of the child with urinary infection. II: Symposium and panel discussion: Problems and advances in diagnosis and management of urinary tract disorders in children. New York J. Med. 64:729-760, 1964.
343. Martius, H.: *Lehrbuch der Gynäkologie*, 2nd ed. Stuttgart, Thieme, 1949.
344. Mathieu, B. J., Goldowsky, S., Chaset, N. and Mathieu, P. L., Jr.: Congenital

deficiency of abdominal muscles with associated multiple anomalies. J. Pediat. 42:92-98, 1953.
345. Meadows, J. A., Jr. and Quattlebaum, R. B.: Polyps of the posterior urethra in children. J. Urol. 100:317-320, 1968.
346. Melick, W. F. and Marizza, J. J.: Renal acidosis and uremia in newborn due to unrecognized bladder neck obstruction. J. Urol. 47:591-601, 1942.
347. Meyer, E.: A new dynamic catheter-type sphincterometer. J. Urol. 90:237-241, 1963.
348. Mijsberg, W. A.: Uber die entwicklung der vagina, des hymen und des sinus urogenitalis beim menschen. Z. Anat. Etwickl. 74:684-760, 1924.
349. Mintz, E. R.: Sarcoma of bladder in children, with report of case. New Eng. J. Med. 205:756-759, 1931.
350. Mitchell, H. C. and Thaemert, J. C.: Three dimensions in fine structure. Science 148:1480-1482, 1965.
351. Mitchell, J. P. and Andrews, G. S.: Clinical aspects and pathology of bladder neck obstruction. Proc. Roy. Soc. Med. 46:549-555, 1953.
352. Mitchell, J. P.: Association of valves in the posterior urethra with bladder neck obstruction. Acta Urol. Belg. 31:507-513, 1963.
353. Mogg, R. A.: Congenital anomalies of the urethra. Brit. J. Urol. 40:638-648, 1968.
354. Moore, V. and Howe, G. E.: Mullerian duct remnants in the male. J. Urol. 70:781-788, 1953.
355. Morales, O. and Romanus, R.: Urethrography in the male with a highly viscous water-soluble contrast medium, Umbradil-Viscous U. Acta Radiol. 95:13-91, 1952.
356. Morgani, G. B.: *Epistola Anatomica Medica.* Liber III, Art, 1751.
357. Morillo, M. M.: Intravesical pressure before and after surgery for bladder neck obstruction. J. Urol. 91:361-363, 1964.
358. Morillo, O. A., Fernandes, M. and Draper, J. W.: Vesicoureteral reflux in male adults with bladder neck obstruction. J. Urol. 89:389-394, 1963.
359. Mostofi, F. K. and Morse, W. H.: Polypoid rhabdomyosarcoma (sarcoma botryoides) of bladder in children. J. Urol. 67:681-687, 1952.
360. Murphy, J. J. and Schoenberg, H. W.: Observations on intravesical pressure changes during micturition. J. Urol. 84:106-110, 1960.
361. Murphy, J. J. and Schoenberg, H. W.: Diagnosis of bladder outlet obstruction. J.A.M.A. 175:354-357, 1961.
362. Murphy, J. J., Schoenberg, H. W. and Tristan, T. A.: Diagnosis and management of lower urinary tract dysfunction in children. J. Urol. 89:192-197, 1963.
363. Muschat, M.: Urethral and perineal cysts of the glands of Cowper. J. Urol. 22:239-246, 1929.
364. McCarthy, J. F., Ritter, J. S. and Klemperer, P.: Anatomical and histological study of the verumontanum with especial reference to the ejaculatory ducts. J. Urol. 17:1-16, 1927.
365. McCrea, E. d'A.: The musculature of the bladder, Proc. Roy. Soc. Med. 19:35-43, 1926.
366. McCrea, L. F.: Congenital valves of the posterior urethra. J. Int. Coll. Surg. 12:342-352, 1949.
367. McDonald, H. P., Upchurch, W. E. and Artime, M.: Bladder dysfunction in children caused by interstitial cystitis. J. Urol. 80:354-356, 1958.
368. McGill, C.: The structure of smooth muscle in the resting and contracted condition. Amer. J. Anat. 9:493-545, 1909.
369. McGovern, J. H. and Marshall, V. F.: Congenital deficiency of the abdominal musculature and obstructive uropathy. Surg. Gynec. Obstet. 108:289-300, 1959.
370. Nanson, E. M.: Marion's disease or bladder neck stenosis. Aust. New Zeal. J. Surg. 20:215-223, 1951.
371. Needham, D. M. and Williams, J. M.: Some properties of uterus actomyosin and myofilaments. Biochem. J. 73:171-181, 1959.

372. Needham, D. M.: Contractile proteins of smooth muscle of the uterus. Physiol. Rev. 42:88-97, 1962.
373. Needham, D. M. and Shoenberg, C. F.: Proteins of the contractile mechanism of mammalian smooth muscle and their possible location in the cell. Proc. Roy. Soc. Med. 160:517-522, 1964.
374. Nesbit, R. M. and Lapides, J.: Tonus of the bladder during spinal "shock." Arch. Surg. 56:138-144, 1948.
375. Nesbit, R. M., Thirlby, R. L. and Raper, F. P.: Diagnosis and treatment of congenital urethral valves. J. Mich. Med. Soc. 50:1244-1247, 1951.
376. Nesbit, R. M. and Baum, W. C.: Diagnosis and management of obstructive uropathy in childhood. Amer. J. Dis. Child. 88:239-250, 1954.
377. Nesbit, R. M. and Crenshaw, W. B.: Treatment of bladder neck contracture by plastic operation. J. Urol. 73:513-519, 1955.
378. Nesbit, R. M.: The genesis of benign polyps in the prostatic urethra. J. Urol. 87:416-418, 1962.
379. Nesbit, R. M., McDonald, H. P., Jr. and Busby, S.: Obstructing valves in the female urethra. J. Urol. 91:79-83, 1964.
380. Neustein, D. H. and Schutte, H.: Müllerian duct cyst, with report of a case. Brit. J. Urol. 40:72-77, 1968.
381. Editorial. Lower urinary tract obstruction in children. New Eng. J. Med. 268:52-53, 1963.
382. Nordenstrom, B. E. W.: Some observations on the shape and course of the female urethra during micturition. Acta Radiol. 38:125-132, 1952.
383. Nunn, I. N.: Bladder neck obstruction in children. J. Urol. 93:693-699, 1965.
384. Nunn, I. N. and Stephens, F. D.: The triad syndrome: A composite anomaly of the abdominal wall, urinary system and testes. J. Urol. 86:782-794, 1961.
385. Obrinsky, W.: Angenesis of abdominal muscles with associated malformation of the genito-urinary tract: case report. Amer. J. Dis. Child. 77:362-373, 1949.
386. Osler, W.: Congenital absence of the abdominal muscles, with distended and hypertrophied urinary bladder. Bull. Hopkins Hosp. 12:331-333, 1901.
387. O'Wilensky, A.: The "mega" syndrome. Amer. J. Med. Sci. 208:602-617, 1944.
388. Pagano, F.: Le valvole congenite dell'uretra. Urologia, 16:64-106, 1965.
389. Panner, B. J. and Honig, C. R.: Filament ultrastructure and organization in vertebrate smooth muscle. Contraction hypothesis based on localization of actin and myosin. J. Cell. Biol. 35:303-321, 1967.
390. Paquin, A. J., Jr., Marshall, V. F. and McGovern, H. H.: The megacystis syndrome. J. Urol. 83:634-646, 1960.
391. Paquin, A. J., Jr., Smith, L. L. and Ochsner, M. G.: Strabismus, ureteral reduplication and megacystis. J. Urol. 87:131-133, 1962.
392. Paquin, A. J.: Surgery of the ureterovesical junction. In Glenn, J. F. and Boyce, W. H.: *Urologic Surgery*. New York, Hoeber, 1969.
393. Parker, R. W.: Case of an infant in whom some of the abdominal muscles were absent. Trans. Clin. Soc. Lond. 28:201, 1895.
394. Patten, B. M.: *Human Embryology*, 2nd ed. New York, McGraw-Hill, 1953.
395. Peachey, L. D. and Porter, K. R.: Intracellular impulse conduction in muscle cells. Science 129:721-722, 1959.
396. Pennington, L. T. and Lund, H. Z.: An elastic ring of tissue in the male urethra: Its probable relationship to primary intrinsic urethral resistance and incontinence following prostatectomy. J. Urol. 84:481-487, 1960.
397. Perlmutter, A. and Retik, A. B.: Long term effects of unilateral vesical denervation in a canine bifid bladder. Invest. Urol. 4:539-545, 1967.
398. Péterfi, P.: Die Muskulatur der Meschlichen Harnblase. Anat. Hefte 50:633, 1914.
399. Petersén, I. and Franksson, C.: Electromyographic study of the striated muscles of the male urethra. Brit. J. Urol. 27:148-153, 1955.
400. Petersén, I., Kjellberg, S. and Dhuner, K. G.: The effect of the intravenous injection of succinylcholine on micturition: An electromyographic study. Brit. J. Urol. 33:392-396, 1961.

401. Pettigrew, J. B.: On the muscular arrangements of the bladder and prostate and the manners in which the ureters and urethra are enclosed. Philosoph. Trans. 157:17-48, 1867.
402. Pierce, J. M., Martyn, G. E. and Roberts, V. L.: Lower urinary tract resistance; pressure-flow relationships. J. Urol. 95:671-673, 1965.
403. Pisani, L.: Sullo sfintere liscio vesicale. Urologia 15:149-153, 1948.
404. Plum, F. and Cofelt, R. H.: The genesis of vesical rhythmicity. Arch. Neurol. 2:487-496, 1960.
405. Pohlman, A. G.: The development of the cloaca in human embryos. Amer. J. Anat. 12:1-26, 1911.
406. Politano, V. A. and Leadbetter, W. F.: An operative technique for the correction of vesicoureteral reflux. J. Urol. 79:932-941, 1958.
407. Politzer, G.: Das schicksal des sinus urogenitalis beim Weibe. Z. Mikr. Anat. Forsch. 59:6-28, 1952.
408. Politzer, G.: Zur normalen und abnormalen entwicklung der menschlichen scheide. Anat. Anz. 102:271-278, 1955.
409. Polse, S. and Edelbrock, H.: Prostatic utricular enlargement as a cause of vesical outlet obstruction in children. J. Urol. 100:329-332, 1968.
410. Porter, K. R. and Palade, G. E.: Studies on the endoplasmic reticulum. III: Its form and distribution in striated muscle cells. J. Biophys. Biochem. Cytol. 3:269-300, 1957.
411. Porter, K. R.: The sarcoplasmic reticulum: Its recent history and present status. J. Biophys. Biochem. Cytol. 10:219-226, 1961.
412. Powell, T. O.: The clinical management of urinary retention in children. J.A.M.A. 153:1341-1346, 1953.
413. Praetorius, G.: Zur pathologie der pars prostatica und der prostata. I. Uber die nicht tuberkulösen stricturer der pars prostatica. Z. Urol. 17:129-146, 1923.
414. Prather, G. C.: *Urological Aspects of Spinal Cord Injuries*. Springfield, Charles C Thomas, 1947.
415. Presman, D.: Congenital valves of the posterior urethra. J. Urol. 86:602-611, 1961.
416. Prosser, C. L., Smith, C. E. and Melton, C. E.: Conduction of action potentials in the ureter of the rat. Amer. J. Physiol. 181:651-660, 1955.
417. Prosser, C. L.: Conduction in non-striated muscles. Proceedings of a symposium on vascular smooth muscle. Physiol. Rev. 42(Suppl. 5): 193-206, 1962.
418. Prosser, C. L.: Introduction to symposium on gastrointestinal smooth muscle. Gastroenterology 49:389-390, 1965.
419. Prosser, C. L.: Conduction in ureteral and other smooth muscles. In *Ureteral Reflux in Children*. Washington, National Academy of Sciences-National Research Council, 1967.
420. Prosser, C. L.: Electrical and mechanical properties of visceral smooth muscles. In *Neurogenic Bladder* (Symposium) (Boyarsky, S., Ed.). Baltimore, Williams and Wilkins, 1967.
421. Pruzanski, W. and Huvos, A. G.: Smooth muscle involvement in primary muscle disease: I. Myotonic dystrophy. Arch. Path. 83:229-233, 1967.
422. Ramachandran, G. N.: Molecular structure of collagen. Int. Rev. Connect. Tissue Res. 1:127-182, 1953.
423. Ramachandran, G. N. and Kartha, G.: Structure of collagen. Nature 174:269-270, 1954.
424. Randall, A.: Median bars as found at autopsy. J. Urol. 1:383-403, 1917.
425. Raper, F. P.: The recognition and treatment of congenital urethral valves. Brit. J. Urol. 25:136-141, 1953.
426. Rattner, W. H., Meyer, R. and Bernstein, J.: Congenital abnormalities of the urinary system. IV. Valvular obstruction of the posterior urethra. J. Pediat. 63:84-94, 1963.
427. Raynaud, A.: Récherches embryologiques de la différenciation sexuelle normale de la souris. Bull. Biol. France Belg., Suppl. 29, 1942.

428. Reger, J. F.: The fine structure of fibrillar network and sarcoplasmic reticulum in smooth muscle cells of the ascaris lumbricoides. J. Cell. Biol. 19:81A, 1963.
429. Rehfisch, E.: Über den mechanismus des harnblasenverschlusses und der harnentleerung. Virchow Arch. Path. Anat. 150:111-151, 1897.
430. Reisman, D. D.: Bladder neck obstructions in children. J.A.M.A. 188:1057-1061, 1964.
431. Reule, G. R. and Ansell, J. S.: Discordant occurrence of genitourinary defects in monozygotic twins. J. Urol. 97:1078-1081, 1967.
432. Richardson, K. C.: Electron microscopic observations on Auerbach's plexus in the rabbit with special reference to the problem of smooth muscle innervation. Amer. J. Anat. 13:99-136, 1958.
433. Richardson, F. H.: External urethroplasty in women; technique and clinical evaluation. J. Urol. 101:719-723, 1969.
434. Rickham, P. P.: Advanced lower urinary obstruction in childhood. Arch. Dis. Child. 37:122-131, 1962.
435. Ritter, R. C., Zinner, N. R. and Paquin, A. J.: Clinical urodynamics. II: An analysis of pressure-flow relations in the normal female urethra. J. Urol. 91:161-165, 1964.
436. Robertson, W. B. and Hayes, J. A.: Congenital diaphragmatic obstruction of the male posterior urethra. Brit. J. Urol. 41:592-598, 1969.
437. Rohner, T. J. and Schoenberg, H. W.: The effect of retropubic revision of the bladder neck upon voiding induced by electrical stimulation. J. Urol. 96:919-920, 1966.
438. Rohner, T. J. and Schoenberg, H. W.: Biochemical comparison of normal and neurogenic animal bladder muscle. I: Changes in glycogen content of dog bladder muscle after spinal cord transection. Invest. Urol. 6:9-15, 1968.
439. Rohner, T. J., Jr., Komins, J., Razlo, N. H. and Schoenberg, H. W.: Biochemical comparison of normal and neurogenic animal bladder muscle. II: Glycogen changes in dog bladder muscle after spinal cord transection and quantitative study. Invest. Urol. 6:16-20, 1968.
440. Rolnick, H. C. and Arnheim, F. K.: An anatomic study of the external urethral sphincter in relation to prostatic surgery. J. Urol. 61:591-603, 1949.
441. Rosenbluth, J.: Smooth muscle: An ultrastructural basis for the dynamics of its contraction. Science 148:1337-1339, 1965.
442. Ross, G., Jr. and Thompson, I. M.: Role of smooth muscle regeneration in urinary tract repair. J. Urol. 95:541-548, 1966.
443. Rothfield, S. H. and Sutton, A. A.: Vesicoureteroplasty combined with Y-V plasty for bladder neck obstruction and secondary reflux: Critical analysis of long term results. J. Urol. 95:197-200, 1966.
444. Rubritius, H. and Schwartz, O.: Contribution to the problem of contracture of the neck of the bladder. J. Urol. 15:461-466, 1926.
445. Rubritius, H.: Die hypertonie des innern blasensphinkters. Urologia 5:185, 1938.
446. Ruch, T. C. and Tang, P. C.: The higher control of the bladder. In *Neurogenic Bladder* (Boyarsky, J., Ed.). Baltimore, Williams and Wilkins, 1967.
447. Rudhe, U.: Roentgenographic diagnosis of obstructive disorders of the lower urinary tract in infants and childhood. Postgrad. Med. J. 35:29-39, 1964.
448. Sabetian, M.: The role of the vesical mucosa in reflex micturition. Brit. J. Urol. 37:417-423, 1965.
449. Sabetian, M.: The genesis of bladder tone. Brit. J. Urol. 37:424-432, 1965.
450. Scheinar, J. and Utikalova, A.: Năse kusenostis YV plastikou hrdla při rozených prouchách vypradnovánimocového měchyře. Rozhl. Chir. 47:737-741, 1968.
451. Scher, S.: Some observations on the anatomy of the bladder neck and posterior urethra with reference to prostatic obstruction. Brit. J. Urol. 22:116-124, 1950.
452. Schwartz, O. and Brenner, A.: Untersuchung uber die physiologie und pathologie der blasenfunktion. VIII. Z. Urol. 32:36-69, 1922.

453. Scott, F. B., Quesada, E. M. and Cardus, D.: Studies on the dynamics of micturition: Observations on healthy men. J. Urol. 92:455-463, 1964.
454. Scott, F. B., Quesada, E. M., Cardus, D. and Laskowski, T.: Electronic bladder stimulation: Dog and human experiments. Invest. Urol. 3:231-243, 1965.
455. Shand, D. G., MacKenzie, J. C., Cattell, W. R. and Cato, J.: Estimation of residual urine volume with I-131 Hippuran. Brit. J. Urol. 40:196-201, 1968.
456. Shoenberg, C. F.: Contractile proteins of vertebrate smooth muscle. Nature 206:526-527, 1965.
457. Shoenberg, C. F.: An electron microscope study of smooth muscle in pregnant uterus of the rabbit. J. Biophys. Biochem. Cytol. 4:609-614, 1958.
458. Shopfner, C. E.: Roentgenologic evaluation of bladder neck obstruction: 527 children. Amer. J. Roentgen. 100:162-176, 1967.
459. Silverman, F. N. and Huang, N.: Congenital absence of abdominal muscles, associated with malformation of the genitourinary and alimentary tracts: Report of cases and review of the literature. Amer. J. Dis. Child. 70:90-124, 1950.
460. Simons, I.: Studies in bladder function. The sphincterometer. J. Urol. 35:96-102, 1936.
461. Simons, I.: Neurologic studies by means of the microcystometer and the sphincterometer. J. Urol.. 39:791-812, 1938.
462. Sleator, W., Jr. and Butcher, H. R., Jr.: Action potentials and pressure changes in ureteral peristaltic waves. Amer. J. Physiol. 180:261-276, 1955.
463. Smith, Blanca de: Pre- and postnatal development of the intramural vesical ganglia in children. Ph.D. thesis, Ohio State University, 1964.
464. Smith, J. C.: Some theoretical aspects of urethral resistance. Invest. Urol. 1:477-481, 1964.
465. Smith, J. C.: Urethral resistance to micturition. Brit. J. Urol. 40:125-156, 1968.
466. Smith, R. D.: The obstructed bladder outlet in childhood. Brit. J. Urol. 34:304-311, 1962.
467. Sole-Balcells, F. and Gosalbez, R.: Valvulas urethrales en la infancia. Arch. Esp. Urol. 19:43-56, 1966.
468. Spellman, R. M. and Kickham, C. J.: Management of the neurogenic bladder in spina bifida. J. Urol. 88:243-244, 1962.
469. Spence, H. M. and Chenoweth, V. C.: Cysts of the prostatic utricle (müllerian duct cysts): Report of two cases in children, each containing calculi, cured by retropubic operation. J. Urol. 79:308-314, 1958.
470. Spence, H. M. and Allen, T.: Congenital absence of abdominal musculature. Urologic aspects. J.A.M.A. 187:814-818, 1964.
471. Stein, J. and Weinberg, S. F.: A histologic study of the normal and dilated ureter. J. Urol. 87:33-38, 1962.
472. Stephens, F. D., Joske, R. A. and Simmons, R. T.: Megaureter with vesicoureteric reflux in twins. Aust. New Zeal. J. Surg. 24:192-194, 1955.
473. Stephens, F. D.: Treatment of megaureters by multiple micturition. Aust. New Zeal. J. Surg. 27:130-134, 1957.
474. Stephens, F. D. and Lenaghan, D.: Anatomical basis and dynamics of vesicoureteral reflux. J. Urol. 87:669-700, 1962.
475. Stephens, F. D.: *Congenital Malformations of the Rectum, Anus and Genito-urinary Tract.* London, Livingstone, 1963.
476. Stöhr, P.: In *Mollendorff's Handbuch der Mikroskop. Anat. des Mensch.* Vol. 4. Berlin, Springer, 1928.
477. Straffon, R. A., Turnbull, R. B. and Mercer, R. D.: The ileal conduit in the management of children with neurogenic lesions of the bladder. J. Urol. 89:198-206, 1963.
478. Stueber, P. J. and Persky, L.: Solid tumors of the urethra and bladder neck. J. Urol. 102:205-209, 1969.
479. Susset, J. G., Rabinovitch, H. and MacKinnon, K. J.: Parameters of micturition: A clinical study. J. Urol. 94:113-221, 1965.

480. Susset, J. G. and Boctor, Z. N.: Implantable electrical vesical stimulator: Clinical experience. J. Urol. 98:673-678, 1968.
481. Suter, F.: Ein beitrag zur histologie und genese der congenitalen divertikel der männlichen harnröhre. Arch. Klin. Chir. 87:225-242, 1908.
482. Swaiman, K. F. and Bradley, W. E.: Maturational biochemical changes in rabbit bladder muscle. Invest. Urol. 5:115-118, 1967.
483. Swenson, O. and Fisher, J. H.: The relation of megacolon and megaloureter. New Eng. J. Med. 253:1147-1150, 1955.
484. Swenson, O., MacMahon, H. E., Jacques, W. E. and Campbell, J. S.: New concept of the etiology of megaloureter. New Eng. J. Med. 246:41-46, 1952.
485. Talbot, H. S. and Bunts, R. C.: Late renal changes in paraplegia; Hydronephrosis due to vesicoureteral reflux. J. Urol. 61:870-880, 1949.
486. Tanagho, E. A. and Pugh, R. C. B.: The anatomy and function of the uretero-vesical junction. Brit. J. Urol. 35:151-165, 1963.
487. Tanagho, E. A. and Smith, D. R.: The anatomy and function of the bladder neck. Brit. J. Urol. 38:54-71, 1966.
488. Tanagho, E. A., Meyers, F. H. and Smith, D. R.: Urethral resistance: Its components and implications. I: Smooth muscle component. Invest. Urol. 7:136-149, 1969.
489. Tanagho, E. A. and Meyers, F. H.: The internal sphincter: Is it under sympathetic control? Invest. Urol. 7:79-89, 1969.
490. Tanagho, E. A., Meyers, F. H. and Smith, D. R.: Urethral resistance: Its components and implications. II: Striated muscle component. Invest. Urol. 7:195-205, 1969.
491. Tang, P-C and Ruch, T. C.: Non-neurogenic basis of bladder tonus. Amer. J. Physiol. 181:249-257, 1955.
492. Taylor, J. S.: Primary dilatation of the bladder neck and urethra in boys. Brit. J. Urol. 41:320-323, 1969.
493. Thaemert, J. C.: An electron microscopic study of smooth muscle. Ph.D. Thesis, University of Colorado, 1959.
494. Thaemert, J. C.: Intercellular bridges as protoplasmic anastomoses between smooth muscle cells. J. Biophys. Biochem. Cytol. 6:67-70, 1959.
495. Thaemert, J. C.: The ultrastructure and disposition of vesiculated nerve processes in smooth muscle. J. Cell Biol. 16:361-377, 1963.
496. Thaemert, J. C.: Ultrastructural interrelationships of nerve processes and smooth muscle cells in three dimensions. J. Cell Biol. 28:37-49, 1966.
497. Thompson, G. J.: Urinary obstruction of the vesical neck and posterior urethra of congenital origin. J. Urol. 47:591-601, 1942.
498. Thompson, G. S.: Note on a case of hydronephrosis with urethral septum causing obstruction to urinary flow. Lancet 1:506, 1907.
499. Timm, G. W. and Bradley, W. E.: Electrostimulation of the urinary detrusor to effect contraction and evacuation. Invest. Urol. 6:562-568, 1969.
500. Tolmatschew, N.: Ein fall von semilunaren klappen der harnröhre und von vergrösserter vesicula prostatica. Arch. Path. Anat. Physiol. 49:348-365, 1870.
501. Torres, H. and Bennett, M. J.: Neurofibromatosis of the bladder: Case report and review of the literature. J. Urol. 96:910-912, 1966.
502. Trabucco, A., Marquez, F. and Pinacci, J.: Endoscopic resection in obstruction of posterior urethra. Rev. Argent. Urol. 17:341-350, 1948.
503. Tristan, T. A., Murphy, J. J. and Schoenberg, H. W.: Cinéfluorographic investigation of genito-urinary tract function: combined, simultaneous and synchronous cinéfluorography and intravesical manometry in evaluation of neurogenic bladder function and bladder outlet obstruction. Radiology 79:731-739, 1962.
504. Truc, E., Grasset, D., Badosa, J., Dossa, J. and Cordier, M.: Ectasic syndrome in a child caused by a polyp of the posterior urethra. J. Urol. Nephrol. 68:812-813, 1962.
505. Tudor, J. M., Carter, O. W. and McClellen, R. E.: An analysis of 2403 consecutive pediatric urological consultations. J. Urol. 87:68-72, 1962.

506. Uhlenhuth, E., Hunter, DeW. T., Jr. and Loechel, W. F.: *Problems in the Anatomy of the Pelvis.* Philadelphia, J. B. Lippincott, 1953.
507. Valdés-Dapena, M. A.: *An Atlas of Fetal and Neonatal Histology.* Philadelphia, J. B. Lippincott, 1957.
508. Velpeau, A. A. L. M.: Urèthre: Cathétérisme. Nouv. Élém. Méd. Opérat. 3:905-911, 1832.
509. Versari, R.: Recherches sur la tunique musculaire de la vessie et spécialement sur le muscle sphinctre interne. Ann. Malad. Organes Genitourin. Part I, 1089-1104, Part II, 1151-1175, 1897.
510. Vilas, E.: Über die entwicklung der menschlichen scheide. Z. Anat. Entwickl. 98:263-292, 1932.
511. Vilas, E.: Über die entwicklung des utriculus prostaticus beim menschen. Z. Anat. Entwickl. 99:599-621, 1933.
512. von Garrelts, B.: Analysis of micturition: A new method of recording the voiding of the bladder. Acta Chir. Scand. 112:326-340, 1957.
513. von Garrelts, B.: Intravesical pressure and urinary flow in normal subjects. Acta Chir. Scand. 114:49-66, 1957-58.
514. von Garrelts, B.: Micturition in the normal male. Acta Chir. Scand. 114:197-210, 1957-58.
515. von Garrelts, B.: Micturition in urethral stricture. Acta Chir. Scand. 114:466-489, 1957-58.
516. von Hösli, P-O.: *Anomalien der Harnwege in Kindesalter und ihre Chirurgische Behandlung.* Basel, S. Karger, 1960.
517. von Lichtenberg, A., Voelcker, F. and Wildbloz, E.: *Handbuch der Urologie,* 5th ed. Berlin, Springer-Verlag. 1928.
518. von Lüdinghausen, H. J. F. H.: Die Anatomischen Grundlagen des Verschlussinechanismus der Weiblichen Harnblase. Z. Anat. Entwickl. 97:757-766, 1932.
519. Waldeyer, W.: Über die sogennante ureterscheide. Anat. Anz., 259-260, 1892.
520. Waldeyer, W.: *Das Trigonum Vesicale.* Berlin, Sitz. Ber. Akad., 1897.
521. Waldeyer, W.: *Das Becken.* Bonn, Fr. Cohen, 1899.
522. Walford, R. L., Moyer, D. L. and Schneider, R. B.: The structure of elastin. Arch. Path. 72:158-165, 1961.
523. Wallace, D. M.: Bladder neck in urinary obstruction. Proc. Roy. Soc. Med. 44:434-437, 1931.
524. Waterhouse, K. and Scordamaglia, L. J.: Anterior urethral valve: A rare cause of bilateral hydronephrosis. J. Urol. 87:556-559, 1962.
525. Waterhouse, K. and Hamm, F. C.: The importance of urethral valves as a cause of vesical neck obstruction in children. J. Urol. 87:404-408, 1962.
526. Waterhouse, K.: The dilated posterior urethra. I. Male. J. Urol. 91:71-75, 1964.
527. Watson, E. M.: The structural basis for congenital valve formation in the posterior urethra. J. Urol. 7:371-381, 1922.
528. Wein, A. J., Gregory, J. G., Sansone, T. C., Rohner, T. J., Jr. and Schoenberg, H. W.: Qualitative studies of the phosphorylase, succinic dehydrogenase, adenosine triphosphatase and glycogen synthetase content of normal, neurogenic and defunctionalized bladder muscle. Invest. Urol. 8:177-181, 1970.
529. Weinberg, S.: Electrophysiology of ureter: Study by extraluminal recording electrode. J. Urol. 91:482-487, 1964.
530. Weinstein, H. J. and Ralph, P. H.: Myofilaments from smooth muscle. Proc. Soc. Exp. Biol. Med. 78:614-615, 1951.
531. Wesson, M. B.: Anatomical, embryological and physiological studies of the trigone and neck of the bladder. J. Urol. 4:279-315, 1920.
532. Weyerbacher, A. F. and Balch, J. F.: Leiomyosarcoma of bladder, with report of case and review of literature. J. Urol. 38:278-287, 1937.
533. Whitaker, J. and Johnston, G. S.: Estimation of urinary outflow resistance in children: Simultaneous measurement of bladder pressure, flow rate and exit pressure. Invest. Urol. 3:379-389, 1966.

534. Whitaker, J., Johnston, G. S. and Lawson, J. D.: Urinary outflow resistance estimation in children. Invest. Urol. 7:127-135, 1969.
535. Williams, D. I.: The development of the trigone of the bladder. Brit. J. Urol. 23:123-128, 1951.
536. Williams, D. I.: The foetal ureter. Brit. J. Urol. 23:336-371, 1951.
537. Williams, D. I.: The chronically dilated ureter. Ann. Roy. Coll. Surg. 14: 107-123, 1954.
538. Williams, D. I.: Congenital bladder neck obstruction and megaureter. Brit. J. Urol. 29:389-392, 1957.
539. Williams, D. I.: Urology in childhood. In *Encyclopedia of Urology*, Vol. 15. Berlin, Springer Verlag, 1958.
540. Williams, D. I. and Schistad, G.: Lower urinary tract tumours in children. Brit. J. Urol. 36:51-65, 1964.
541. Williams, D. I. and Eckstein, H. B.: Obstructive valves in the posterior urethra. J. Urol. 93:236-246, 1965.
542. Williams, D. I. and Abbassian, A.: Solitary pedunculated polyp of the posterior urethra in children. J. Urol. 96:483-486, 1966.
543. Williams, D. I. and Burkholder, G. V.: The prune-belly syndrome. J. Urol. 98:244-259, 1967.
544. Williams, D. I.: *Paediatric Urology*. New York, Appleton, Century, Crofts, 1968.
545. Williams, D. I. and Retik, A. B.: Congenital valves and diverticula of the anterior urethra. Brit. J. Urol. 41:228-234, 1969.
546. Williams, D. I. and Taylor, J. S.: A rare congenital uropathy; vesico-urethral dysfunction with upper tract anomalies. Brit. J. Urol. 41:307-313, 1969.
547. Wilson, M. C., Horton, G. R., Horton, B. F. and Byrne, J. W.: Retropubic approach to bladder neck resection in children. Arch. Surg. 68:87-92, 1954.
548. Winckler, G.: Contribución al estudio de la inervación de las visceras pelvianas. Arch. Esp. Urol. 20:259-279, 1967.
549. Winckler, G.: L'innervation des vicères pelviens chez le mouton: participation du nerf honteux interne. Arch. Anat. 40:85-89, 1967.
550. Winter, C. C.: Radioisotope uroflometry and bladder residual test. J. Urol. 91:103-106, 1964.
551. Wolgin, W., Rosenberg, M. and Muschat, M.: Coexistence of congenital median bar and urethral valves. J. Urol. 68:506-509, 1952.
552. Wolinsky, H. and Glagov, S.: Structural basis for the static mechanical properties of the aortic media. Circ. Res. 14:400-413, 1964.
553. Woodburne, R. T.: Structure and function of the urinary bladder. J. Urol. 84:79-85, 1960.
554. Woodburne, R. T.: The sphincter mechanism of the urinary bladder. Anat. Rec. 141:11-20, 1961.
555. Woodburne, R. T.: The ureter, ureterovesical junction, and vesical trigone. Anat. Rec. 151:243-249, 1965.
556. Young, B. W.: The retropubic approach to vesical neck obstruction in children. Surg. Gynec. Obstet. 96:150-154, 1953.
557. Young, B. W. and Goebel, J. L.: Retropubic wedge excision in congenital vesical neck obstruction. Stanford Med. Bull. 12:106-123, 1954.
558. Young, B. W., Anderson, W. J. and King, G. G.: Radiographic estimation of residual urine in children. J. Urol. 75:263-272, 1956.
559. Young, B. W. and Niebel, J. D.: Vesico-urethroplasty for congenital vesical neck obstruction in children. J. Urol. 79:838-843, 1958.
560. Young, B. W.: Elastic components of the vesical neck and urethra in childhood. Invest. Urol. 3:20-32, 1965.
561. Young, B. W.: Die anatomischen grundlagen fur die vesicourethroplastik. Verh. Deutsch. Ges. Urol. 22:95-97, 1969.
562. Young, H. H.: A new procedure (punch operation) for small prostatic bars and contracture of the prostatic orifice. J.A.M.A. 40:253-257, 1913.

563. Young, H. H., Frontz, W. A. and Baldwin, J. C.: Congenital obstruction of the posterior urethra. J. Urol. 3:289-354, 1919.
564. Young, H. H. and Cash, J. R.: A case of pseudohermaphrodismus masculinus, showing hypospadias, greatly enlarged utricle, abdominal testis and absence of seminal vesicles. J. Urol. 5:405-430, 1921.
565. Young, H. H. and Wesson, M. B.: The anatomy and surgery of the trigone. Arch. Surg. 3:1-37, 1921.
566. Young, H. H. and McKay, R. W.: Congenital valvular obstruction of prostatic urethra. Surg. Gynec. Obstet. 48:509-535, 1929.
567. Youngblood, V. H., Tomlin, E. M. and Crosland, D. B.: Contracture of bladder neck: Experience with Bradford Young operation. Southern Med. J. 51:1516-1522, 1958.
568. Zangemeister, W.: Verschluss der weiblichen blase. Z. Gynak. Urol. 1:79-81, 1908.
569. Zapp, E.: *Neue Pädiatrische Urologie*. Stuttgart, Ferdinand Enke Verlag, 1960.
570. Zatz, L. M.: Combined physiologic and radiologic studies of bladder function in female children with recurrent urinary tract infections. Invest. Urol. 3:278-308, 1965.
571. Zinner, N. R. and Paquin, A. J., Jr.: Clinical urodynamics. I: Studies of intravesical pressure in normal human female subjects. J. Urol. 90:719-730, 1963.
572. Zinner, R., Ritter, R. C., Sterling, A. M. and Harding, D. C.: High-speed cinematography of human urination. Invest. Urol. 6:605-610, 1969.

Index

Page numbers followed by f indicate figures.

Abscess(es), 150
Acetylcholine, 81
Acetylcholinesterase, 53
Achalasia, 131
Actin, 77, 78, 81
Action potential(s), 80, 81, 82
Adenoma(s), 93
    prostatic, 5
Adenosine triphosphate, 77, 83
Adenosine triphosphatase, 77, 82
Adventitia, 51, 143, 148
Aganglionosis, 147
Agenesis, renal, 155
Aging, 83
    response of muscles to, 117
    tissue balance and, 58
Albarran, J., 39
    sphincter of, 45
Aldolase, 136
Alken, C. E., 7
Allantois, 15
Amino acid(s), 83, 84, 85
Amyotonia, 95
Amyotonic dystrophy, 134
Anastomosis, ureteroureterocutaneous, 166
Anderson, W. J., 149
Anemia, 154
Anesthesia, 157, 159
Ansell, J. S., 103

Antibacterial therapy, 160, 164, 166
Aorta, 48
Aplasia of penis, 4
Arc(s), Pennington's, 45, 66, 115
    transverse precervical, 30, 31, 33, 45, 67
Arey, L. B., 126
Arnheim, F. K., 33
Artery(ies), 139
    hypogastric, 23
    iliac, 20
    inferior vesical, 20
    pudendal, 20
    superior vesical, 19
    supply to bladder of, 19–20, 21f
    vesiculodeferential, 20
Atropine, 79
Autonomic nervous system, 48, 133
Axon(s), 50, 79, 82

Balance, detrusor-sphincter, 95, 96, 131, 134
    as surgical guide, 160
    urinary-tract, 161
Baldwin, J. C., 7, 8, 98, 100
Bandelette(s), 31. *See also* Bundle(s), posterior longitudinal
Barkow, H. C., 10
Barr, L. A., 82

Index **191**

Barrett, G. S., 142
Bartholin's duct(s), 3, 16
Bazy, M., 9
Beach, P. D., 130
Beer, E., 6
Bell, C., 36
Benavent, C., 116
Bengmark, S., 15
Bergman, R. A., 58, 76, 77
Bevans, M., 134
Bio-assay, 135
Bladder(s), 143
  anatomy of, 11-63
  capacity of, 95
  contracted, 134
  development of, 11-19
  filling of, 68f, 75
    normal, 67
  functions of, 76, 146
  gross anatomy of, 23-55
  histotopographic anatomy of, 30-55
  hypertrophy of, 122, 123f, 126, 151
  hypotonic, 145
  innervation of, 48
  megacystitis and, 131
  microscopic anatomy of, 55-63
  musculature of, 23-63
  neurogenic, 81, 82, 146-149, 147f, 148f, 154, 157, 166
  overdistention of, 133, 142
  sarcoma of, 150
  spasms of, 153
  stimulation of, 160
  tonus of, 74, 134
Blinn, K., 74
Blockade(s), neuromuscular, 160
  pudendal, 160
Blood urea nitrogen, 155
Bloomfield, A., 126
Bodian, M., 6, 7, 116, 120, 133
Bone(s), pubic, 26
Bonnet, P., 9
Bonney, V., 86
Bonnin, N. J., 94
Borm, D., 6
Bors, E., 24, 65, 74, 146
Bottaccini, M. R., 86
Boyarsky, S., 80, 146
Bozler, E., 79, 80
Bracci, U., 9
Bradley, W. F., 80, 81, 82, 135
Braithwaite, J. L., 20
Brenner, A., 86
Bro-Rasmussen, F., 24
Bruton, O. C., 142
Brynes, C. K., 131

Bulmer, D., 16, 17, 105
Bundle(s). 28, 29. *See also* Fiber(s); Muscle bundle(s)
  anterior longitudinal, 30, 67
  circular, 27
  detrusor, 33
  fiber, 27
  inner anterior longitudinal, 30, 67
  lateral longitudinal, 36
  paired lateral, 30
  paired posterolateral longitudinal, 31
  posterior, 46
  posterolateral longitudinal, 33, 67
  posterior longitudinal, 31, 33, 67
  post-trigonal, 46
  pubovesical, 23, 24, 26, 30, 75
  smooth-muscle, 23, 24. *See also* Smooth muscle, bundles of
  submucosal longitudinal, 33
Bunting, C. H., 134
Burkholder, G. V., 142, 143
Burns, E., 94
Busby, S., 103
Byrnes, C. K., 78

CAESAR, R., 58, 76, 77
"Camera retrohimenal," 16
Campbell, M. F., 7, 116
Canal(s), vesicourethral, 14f, 15
Cardiomyopathy, 134
Cardus, D., 89
Cash, J. R., 129
Catheter(s), 86, 88
Cauda equina, 146, 167
Caulk, J. R., 6
Ceccarelli, F. E., 130
Cell(s), adrenergic, 53, 73
  cholinergic, 53, 73
  intermediate, 53
Cellule(s), 116
Central nervous system, 79, 142
Chetwood, C. H., 6
Chou, S., 135
Chromatin, 56, 77
Chwalla, R., 7
Cinecystourethrography, 131, 156, 164
  voiding, 121
Cinematography, 89
Cineradiography, 27, 87, 156
Clausen, E., 6
Cloaca, 11, 12, 13f, 15
Cloacal membrane(s). *See* Membrane(s), cloacal
Colic, ureteral, 153

192   Index

Collagen, 55, 56, 58, 59, 60–63, 69, 79, 83–84, 85, 107, 117, 122, 134, 135, 139, 143, 148
Comar, A. E., 146
Conduction, 80
Connective tissue bridge(s), 65
Continence, 10, 64, 67. *See also* Incontinence
 partial, 161
 resting, 66, 76
Contraction, 79
 detrusor and, 81, 82
 mechanism of, 78
 smooth muscle and, 81, 83, 85, 141
Convulsion(s), 153
Conway, C. J., 81
Cook, F. E., 126
Cord(s), sacral, 75, 149, 167
 spinal, 75, 131, 146
Corium, 55, 60, 61
Coronal sulcus, 19, 125
Corpora cavernosa, 50
Corpus spongiosum, 50, 125
Cortical demand, 75
Cowper, William, 126
Cowper's duct(s), 3, 16, 18f, 45, 101f, 102f, 125
 cysts of, 4, 126–128, 128f, 129f, 130f
 defects of, 96
Cowper's gland, 39
Creatine phosphate, 83
Creatine phosphokinase, 82, 136
Creatinine, 155
Crenshaw, W. B., 6
Crista urethralis, 39, 48, 61, 98, 99, 105. *See also* Plicae colliculi
 abnormalities of, 103
Crystalluria, 154
Curare, 65
Cussen, L. J., 134
Cyst(s), 4, 126–130
 congenital, 96, 125
 urachal, 157
Cystic disease, 154
Cystine, 84
Cystitis, 117, 140, 164
 interstitial, 134
 repair in, 121f
Cystitis cystica, 164
Cystography, 131, 155
Cystometrogram(s), 131
Cystometry, voiding, 85, 87, 91
Cystoplasty, reduction, 160
Cystoscopy, 130, 131, 133, 155, 159, 164
Cystourethrocele(s), 89
Cystourethrogram(s), 67
 retrograde, 118f, 119f
 voiding, 70f, 71f, 72f, 106f, 122, 145, 156
Cystourethrography, voiding, 105, 117, 130, 147, 155, 157
Cystourethroscopy, 157
Cytolemma, 56, 78, 139
Cytoplasm, 56

Davies, J., 17
Decompensation, detrusor and, 157
Dell'Adami, G., 9
DeLuca, F. G., 131
"Demilunes," 27
"Demi-valvules," 8
Denny-Brown, D., 64
Denonvilliers' fascia, 22
Dermatitis, ammoniacal, 154
 urinary, 149
Detrusor, 19, 23, 51, 80, 146, 147
 adaptation of, 91
 age-specific variations in, 5
 arterial supply to, 20
 balance with sphincter of, 95, 96, 131, 134
 cells in, 74f
 contraction of, 69, 71f, 81, 82
 decompensation of, 157
 dysfunction of, 157
 dysplasia of, 133
 elastic fibers in, 60
 electrical activity of, 81
 excitation of, 81
 function of, 80
 hypertrophy of, 93, 117, 122
 hypotonia of, 82, 95, 131, 133, 143, 146
 imbrication of, 160
 maturation of, 163
 megacystis and, 133
 muscle bundles in, 24, 28, 29, 67
 musculature of, 25f
 repair of, 121f
 smooth muscle of, 57f
 smooth muscle origins in, 65
 stimulation of, 75
 tonus of, 74
Detrusor imbalance, 58
Detrusor loop(s), 26f, 28, 28f, 31, 33, 35f, 45, 46, 48, 66, 69, 75, 76, 105
 division of, 122
Dewey, M. M., 82
Dhuner, K. G., 65
Diagnosis, 152–159

Diagnostic investigation, 155–159
Diaphragm(s), 98. *See also* Valve(s)
  urethral, 99f
  urogenital, 19, 22, 53
Diffusion theory of excitation, 79
Dilatation, 131
Disease, 83
  tissue components and, 58
Disse, J., 9
"Distal urethral stenosis," 149
Distention, 58
  smooth muscle and, 141
Diversion, ileal-loop, 166
  urinary, 149, 165, 167
Diverticulum(a), 116, 146, 147, 148
  bulbous urethra and, 96
  urethral, 125–126
Dogiel, A. S., 51
Donahue, J. P., 85
Dossot, O., 6, 8
Double voiding, 165
Downs, R. A., 122
Duct(s), 3
  Bartholin's, 3, 16
  Cowper's. *See* Cowper's duct(s)
  ejaculatory, 61
  mesonephric. *See* Mesonephric duct(s)
  müllerian. *See* Müllerian duct(s)
  wolffian, 9, 12, 15, 96, 100
Dysplasia, 148
  muscular, 133
  smooth muscle and, 95
  vesical, 141–146
Dysrhaphia, 95, 147, 167
Dystrophy, amyotonic, 134
  muscular, 134
Dysuria, 153

EAGLE, J. F., Jr., 142
Eberth, C. J., 10
Eckstein, H. B., 146
Edema, inflammatory, 150
  urethral, 164
Edling, N. P. G., 125, 126
Edwards, G. A., 58, 76
Ejaculation, 61, 65, 73, 117
Elastin, 84–85, 117, 122, 134, 135, 148.
  See also Fiber(s), elastic
"Elastomucin," 84
Elastosis, 120, 136, 139, 143
El-Badawi, A., 51, 53
Elbogen, A., 126
Electrical silence, 88

Electrocoagulation, 158
Electrolyte(s), 155
Electromyography, 64, 87, 146
Electron microscopy, 58, 60, 76, 77, 83, 84, 131
Elliott, T. R., 64
Emmet, J. L., 94
Endoplasmic reticulum, 77
Endoscopy, 86, 155, 157, 158, 159
End-plates, motor, 50
Englisch, J., 128
Enhorning, G., 89
Enuresis, 145, 153, 165
Enzyme study(ies), 82, 136
Epididymis, 134, 155
Epinephrine, 81
Epispadias, 166
Epithelium, 53, 55, 161
  prostatic, 123
  squamous metaplasia of, 123
  vaginal, 17
Ericsson, H. O., 17
Erythema, trigonal, 164
Evaluation(s), yearly, of patient, 165
Examination(s), of patient, 153
  rectal, 130, 155
Excitation, detrusor and, 81
  smooth muscle and, 82
Expulsive force(s), 85
Exstrophy, 166

FELIX, W., 16
Fever(s), 153
Fiber(s). *See also* Bundle(s); Muscle bundle(s)
  cervicourethral, 30
  cholinergic, 53
  circular detrusor, 31
  collagen. *See* Collagen
  distribution of, 56–58
  elastic, 39, 58, 59, 60–63, 62f, 69, 79, 84–85, 107, 116, 117, 120f, 139, 141, 148. *See also* Elastin
  levator ani, 39
  plexiform, 31
  posterior (bandelette), 60
  prostatourethral, 36, 38f, 48, 55, 69, 99
  replacement, 140
  sub-sphincteric arc, 36
  vascular, 69
  vesicocervical, 8, 27, 30, 33, 35, 36, 45, 46, 47f, 55, 69

Fiber(s) (*Continued*)
    vesicoprostatourethral, 31, 36, 41, 46
    vesicourethral, 46, 69
Fibroelastosis, 7, 94, 116-120, 148, 149
Fibrosclerosis, 8
Fibrosis, 94, 116, 135, 139, 143, 148
    irreparable, 161
    submucous, 7
Finkle, A. L., 116
Fisher, J. H., 133
Fistula(e), rectourethral, 155
    rectovesical, 155
    umbilical, 142
Flow rate(s), 87, 90f, 92
    decreased, 91
    measurements of, 88
    normal, 156
        maximal, 89
Fluid energy loss, 86
Fluid intake, 153, 164, 165
Fluid loss, 153
Foreign body(ies), 157
Forsberg, J. G., 16
Frazer, J. E., 15, 126
Fredericks, C. M., 81
Frequency, urination and, 154
Frolich, F., 142
Frontz, W. A., 7, 8, 98, 100
Fuchs, N., 100
Fuller, E., 6

GANGLION(A), 51, 53, 73, 74f, 139, 140f, 141, 143, 148
    adventitial, 51, 52f
    autonomic, 50
    deficiency of, 142
    megacystis and, 133
    perivesical, 49
    vesical, 51
    vesical neck and, 50, 50f
Gansler, H., 76, 77
Gastrointestinal tract, 142
    symptom(s) of, 153
Genetic aspects of disease, 136
Genetic fault(s), 103
Gersuny procedure, 166
Gil Vernet, S., 8, 10, 16, 24, 26, 30, 31, 33, 36, 39, 45, 55, 126, 127
    histotopographic anatomy of, 28-29
Gireaux, B., 33
Gland(s), bulbo-urethral, 126
    Cowper's, absence of, 126
Glans penis, 19

Gleason, D. M., 86
Glingar, A., 7
Glomerulonephritis, 154
Glycine, 84
Glycogen, 82, 133
Goebel, J. L., 117
Golgi complex(es), 77
Gomez-Oliveros, L., 10
Graft(s), seromuscular, 160
"Grapple plaque(s)," 78, 131
Gross, R. E., 7, 116
Growth, 160, 161
    kidneys and, 163, 164, 166
    normal, failure of, 154
"Growth lag," 164
Gruenwald, P., 14, 100
Guthrie, G. J., 6
Guyon, J. C. F., 6
    meatus of, 45, 100
Gyllensten, L., 15, 115

HAINES, R. W., 39
Hand, J. R., 94
Harding, D. C., 89
Harman, J. W., 78, 131
Harper, R. C., 143
Harrow, B. R., 131, 133
Hayes, J. A., 98
Headstream, J. W., 131
Heiss, R., 9, 10, 33
Heitz-Boyer-Hovelacque procedure, 166
Hemangioma(s), 151
Hematuria, 153, 154
Hemholz, H. F., 94
Henle, J., 9, 10
Henley, W. L., 133, 142
Hennig, R., 10
Hip(s), dislocation of, 142
Hippuran, 155
Hirschsprung's disease, 95, 133
Histidine, 84
History(ies), of patient, 85, 136, 153
Holm, H. H., 89
Honig, C. R., 76, 78
Hormonal change(s), 103
Horseshoe(s), 27, 33
Howard, F. S., 129
Howe, G. E., 130
Huang, N., 142
Hufeisen, 27
Hunter, DeW. T., Jr., 23, 24, 26, 30
Hutch, J. A., 24, 27, 65, 75, 117
Huvos, A. G., 134

Hydrodynamics, 85-92, 121
Hydromucocolpos, 150
Hydronephrosis, 116, 154, 155, 166
Hydroureteronephrosis, 126
Hydroxyproline, 83
Hyman, A., 133, 142
Hymen(s), 17, 19
  formation of, 105
  imperforate, 100
Hymenal ring(s), 19, 100, 107, 150
Hyperchromatism, 141
Hypereosinophilia, 134
Hyperpolarization, 81
Hypertrophy, 160, 163
  bladder and, 122, 123f, 126, 151
  detrusor and, 93, 117, 122
  smooth muscle and, 58
Hypogastric plexus, 21, 48, 49f, 73, 75, 147
  histotopography of, 48-53
Hypoplasia, 155
Hypospadias, 129
Hypothalamus, 75
Hypotonia, 146, 147
  detrusor and, 82, 95, 131, 133, 143, 146

"IDIOPATHIC vesical neck obstruction," 5
Ikeda, K., 143
Imbrication, detrusor and, 160
Imperforate anus, 155
Incontinence, 65, 146, 154. *See also* Continence
  alleviation of, 160
  stress, 145
Infection(s), 116, 125, 129, 130, 147, 149, 151, 154, 156, 164, 165, 166
  chronic, 161
  uncontrollable, 167
Inferior pubic rami, 22
Inferior vena cava, 20
Inflammation(s), 8, 116, 134, 149
Inhibition, central, 75
  freedom from, 75
  intrinsic striated sphincter and, 76
  reciprocal, 64
  reflex, 75
Innervation, bladder and sphincteric urethra and, 48
  smooth muscle and, 85
    nerves and, 73
  sphincteric system and, 73
  striated muscle and, 39
  sympathetic, of trigone, 64

Innsbruck, University of, 107
Integument(s), 143
Interureteric ridge, 21, 31, 36, 60
Ionic flux, 81
Ischemia, 141

JOHNSON, F. P., 125, 126
Johnston, G. S., 87, 89
Jones, B. W., 131
Jones, H. W., Jr., 17
Junction(s), bulbomembranous, 4
  dorsal urethrovesical, 81
  penoscrotal, 125
  tight, 82
  ureterovesical, 91, 92
    incompetence of, 156
    maturation of, 163
    reconstruction of, 160
  urethrovesical, 33, 82
  vesicourethral, 48
Junctional zone(s), 139, 140

KALISCHER, O., 10, 26, 30, 39
Kartha, G., 83
Kaudelzapfen, 16
Kauffman, J. J., 89
Keitzer, W. A., 116
Kidney(s), 143, 145
  growth of, 163, 164, 166
  hypertrophy of, 163
  infection of, 164
King, G. G., 149
King, L. R., 88, 145
Kjellberg, S. R., 17, 65
Klemperer, P., 61
Knox, J. H., Jr., 100
Koff, A., 16, 17
Kohlrausch, O., 9
Krahn, H. P., 65
Kuntz, A., 51
Kusama, H., 17

LABIA majora, 53, 154
Langenbeck, B. R. K. von, 8
Langer, C. R. von Edenberg, 9
Langer-Toldt, D. T., 10
Langworthy, O. R., 64
Lansing, A. E., 84
Lapides, J., 24, 65, 74, 146
Lattimer, J. K., 86, 142
Lawson, J. D., 87
Leadbetter, G. W., Jr., 85, 122
Leadbetter, W. F., 122

Learmonth, J. R., 64
Lebreton, P., 126
L'Egenbrodt, 8
Legueu, F., 6, 7
Leibowitz, S., 133
Lenaghan, D., 36, 133
Lesion(s), congenital obstructive, pathology of, 93-151. See also specific structures
Leukocyte(s), 139, 140, 154
Lich, R., Jr., 94
Lichtenstein, B. W., 142
Ligament(s), puboprostatic, 23
  pubovaginal, 23
  pubovesical, 30
  triangular, 143
Light microscopy, 1, 58, 60, 77, 122, 135
Lipiodol, 149, 156, 157
"Lissophincter," 9, 10
Loechel, William, 23, 24
Lowsley, O. S., 100
Lund, H. Z., 61, 63
Lyon, R. P., 149

MACROPHAGE(s), 139, 140, 141
Management, 152-167. See also Surgical procedures; Treatment
  definition of, 167
  further considerations in, 161-167
  medical, 161, 164
Manley, C. B., Jr., 24, 39
Marberger, H., 24
Marion, G., 6, 7, 8, 39, 120
Mark, J. S. T., 58, 76, 77, 78
Markland, C., 135
Marshall, V. F., 131, 133
Martius, H., 10
Maturation, 161
  detrusor and, 163
  ureterovesical junctions and, 163
Maurer, J. E., 94
McArdle's disease, 133
McCarthy, J. F., 61
McCrea, E. d'A., 10, 39
McDonald, H. P., Jr., 103, 134
McGovern, H. H., 131, 133
McKay, R. W., 8
McPhee, V. G., 116
Meatus, of Guyon, 45, 100
  urethral. See Urethral meatus
Meconium, 154
Megacolon, 131
Megacystis, 95, 130-141, 142, 145
Megaduodenum, 131

Megaesophagus, 131
Megagastrium, 131
Megalo-urethra, 125
"Megatrigone," 133
Megaureter(s), 133, 135
Mellens, H. Z., 88
Membrane(s), anal, 11
  cloacal, 9, 11, 12f, 100, 105
    failure of, 4
  nuclear, 56
  plasma, 59f, 78, 79
  urogenital, 11
Menarche, 163
Mercier's bar, 36. See also Interureteric ridge
Méry, 126
Mesodermal septum, 17
Mesonephric duct(s), 12, 13, 13f, 14, 15
Mesonephros, 3, 130
Metanephros, 13f
Metaplasia, squamous, of epithelium, 123
Micromanometer(s), 86
Micturition, 24, 153. See also Urination; Voiding
  muscular mechanisms of, 64-73
  neuromuscular mechanisms of, 73-76
  physiology of, 64-92
  pressures in, 87
    changes in, 86
  smooth-muscle bundles and, 27
  straining and, 155
  time of, 87
Midbrain, 75
Mitochondrion(a), 77, 79
Mogg, R. A., 142
Moore, V., 130
Morales, P. A., 65
Morgagni, G. B., 8
Mosely, R. L., 51
Mucosa, 139, 148
  transitional cell, 19
Müller's tubercle, 15
Müllerian duct(s), 3, 9, 14-15, 16, 17, 96, 100, 101f
  cysts of, 128-130
Muscle(s), abdominal, absence of, 95, 133, 142
  amount of, in ureter, 135
  bulbocavernosus, 53, 66, 73
  cardiac, 74, 134
  detrusor. See Detrusor
  expulsive, 66
  intrinsic striated, 39-41, 46, 65
    elastic fibers in, 61-63
  ischiocavernosus, 53, 66, 73

Muscle(s) (*Continued*)
  levator ani, 23, 53, 66
  perineal, 23, 53, 65, 66, 88
    electrical silence in, 64
  rectourethralis, 39
  response to aging of, 117
  retentive, 66
  smooth. *See* Smooth muscle(s)
  striated, 23, 24, 79, 134, 160
    in perineum, 73
  surgical weakening of, 160
  trigonal, 31, 33, 36, 37f, 39, 55, 98
    absence of, 133
    fiber pattern in, 60
    mucosa in, 61
  vesicourethral, in the female, 46-48
Muscle bundle(s), 3. *See also* Bundle(s); Fiber(s)
  distribution of, 22f
  isolation of, 139
  rupture of, 133, 140
Muscular dystrophy, 134
Myasthenia gravis, 134
Myelin, 50
Myelodysplasia, 95, 131, 146
Myelomeningocele(s), 95, 122, 131, 146, 166
Myoblast(s), 140
Myofibril(s), 56, 77, 78, 79, 139, 150
Myopathy, 141
Myosin, 77, 78, 81, 131

NANSON, E. M., 6
Neoplasm(s), renal, 154
Nephrostomy, 165
Nerve(s), 54f, 140f, 148
  autonomic, 74f
  deficit in supply of, 131
  dorsal, of penis, 53
  extrinsic, 80
  intrinsic, 80
  parasympathetic, 133
  perineal, 39, 53
  pudendal, 39, 53-55, 65
    blockade of, 65
    histotopography of, 48-53
    resection of, 160
  smooth muscle innervation and, 73
  somatic, 39
    lesions of, 146
Nerve block(s), pudendal, 65
Nerve bundle(s), 139, 141
Nerve ending(s), 56, 73, 79, 140
  in trigone, 74, 74f
  in vesical neck, 74

Nervi erigentes, 48
Nervous system(s), autonomic, 48, 133
  central, 79, 142
Nesbit, R. M., 6, 74, 103, 123, 146
Neuroblast(s), 51
Neurofibroma(s), 151
Neurogenic bladder. *See* Bladder, neurogenic
Neuromuscular blockade, 160
Neustein, D. H., 128, 130
Nexus(i), 82
Nissl substance, 51
Norepinephrine, 53
Nucleus, nucleoli, 56, 77, 139, 140
  of smooth muscle cell, 77
Nunn, I. N., 88, 133

OBSERVATION of patient, 85, 164
Odor, urine and, 153, 154
O'Hegarty, M. T., 78, 131
Orifice(s), fistulous, 157
  hymenal, 17
  internal, 27
  ureteral, 51, 95, 164
    ectopic, 157
  ureterovesical, 36
  urethral, 33, 73
  vaginal, 159
Osler, William, 141
Overdistention, bladder and, 142
O'Wilensky, A., 131

PAGANO, R., 9
Pain, 74, 153, 154
Palade, G. E., 79
Panner, B. J., 76, 78
Paquin, A. J., 90, 131, 133
Paramyosin, 78
Parker, R. W., 142
Pattern(s), pressure, 156
  urinary, 155, 163
  voiding, obstructed, 117
Peachy, L. D., 79
Pectus excavatum, 142
Penis, aplasia of, 4
Pennington, L. T., 61, 63
Pennington's arc, 45, 66, 115
Perimysium, 139
Perineum, 23, 66, 155
  striated muscle in, 73
Periosteum, 22
Peterfi, P., 9
Petersen, I., 65
"Petits tendons," 33, 60

Pettigrew, J. B., 10
Phallus, 19
Phosphorylase, 82, 133
Pink urine, 153
Pinocytotic vesicle(s), 77
Pinworm(s), 154
Pisani, L., 7
Plexus(es), hypogastric. *See* Hypogastric plexus
  neuroterminal, 53
  pelvic, 48
  perivascular, 53
  perivesical, 50, 73
  of Santorini, 20
Plica(e), inframontane mucosal, 9
Plicae colliculi, 9, 18f, 19, 98, 104f. *See also* Crista urethralis
Plication, vesical, 160
Pneumaturia, 154
Politzer, G., 16
Polyp(s), 96
  urethral, 122–125, 124f
Porter, K. R., 79
Pouch, rectal, 166
Powell, T. O., 142
Praetorius, G., 6
Prather, G. C., 146
Precervical arc, 30, 31, 33, 45, 67
Pressure(s), changes in, in micturition, 86
  intra-abdominal, 89
  intra-urethral, 88
  intravesical, 86, 88, 91, 92, 131
  measurements of, 88
  micturition, 87
  patterns of, 156
  postmicturition, 87
  resting, 87, 91, 92
  voiding, 89, 91
Pressure flow measurement(s), 85
Pressure gradient(s), 86, 88, 89
Progesterone, 103
Proline, 83, 84
Prosser, C. L., 79, 80, 82
Prostate(s), 5, 20, 22, 26, 31, 33, 38, 41, 45, 48, 56, 73, 134
  sarcoma of, 150
  transurethral resection of, 94
Prostatic utricle(s), 17
Prune-belly syndrome. *See* Triad syndrome
Pruzanski, W., 134
Pseudoelastin, 84, 120
Pubic bone, 26
Pubis, 24
Puboprostatic ligament(s), 23
Pubovaginal ligament(s), 23
Pubovesical bundle(s), 23, 24, 26, 30
Pubovesical ligament(s), 30
Pudendal block, 160
Pyelography, 155
Pyelonephritis, 164, 166
Pyknosis, 141
Pyuria, 153, 154

Queseda, E. M., 89

Radiography, 86
  urogenital sinus and, 159
Radioisotope(s), 86
Radioisotope uroflowmetry, 92
Ralph, P. H., 76
Ramachandran, G. N., 83
Randell, A., 6
Randolph, J., 7, 116
Raynaud, A., 17
Reciprocal inhibition, 64
Rectal pouch, 166
Rectosigmoid, 143
Rectourethralis confluence, 66
Rectum, 11, 21, 22
Red urine, 154
Reflux, prevention of, 160
  ureteral, 91, 92, 95, 131, 132f, 133, 145, 147, 156
  vaginal, 72f, 165
Reger, J. F., 79
Rehfisch, E., 86
Relaxation, 79, 82
Renal agenesis, 155
Renal failure, 126, 167
Renal scanning, 155
Renal transplantation, 165
Resection, transurethral, 39, 94, 122, 159
Residual urine, 93, 131, 142, 145, 146, 154, 156, 157, 158f, 161
  elimination of, 160
Resistance(s), 85
  sphincters and, 86
    reduction of, 160
  sphincteric urethra and, 86, 122
  urethral, 91, 92, 156
    calculation of, 88
    normal, 87
Resting potential(s), 80
Retik, A. B., 125
Retropubic approach, 94
Retzius, space of, 21

Reul, G. R., 103
Rhabdomyosarcoma(s), 150, 151
Rhythmicity, 74
Ribonucleic acid, 77
Rigidity, 141, 149, 150
Ritter, J. S., 61
Ritter, R. C., 89, 90
Robertson, E. G., 64
Robertson, W. B., 98
Rohner, T. J., 133
Rolnick, H. C., 24, 33
Rosenbluth, J., 78
Rubritius, H., 6, 7, 10
Rudhe, U., 17, 122
Ruska, H., 58, 76

SABETIAN, M., 74
Sacral cord, 75, 149, 167
Sacral promontory, 48
Santorini, plexus of, 20
Sarcoma, 150
Sarcomere(s), 78
Sarcoplasm, 77, 140
Sarcoplasmic reticulum, 79
Sarcotubule(s), 79
Scanning, renal, 155
Schenk, E. A., 51, 53
Scher, S., 133
Schutte, H., 128, 130
Schwartz, O., 7, 86
Scott, F. B., 89
Scott, W. W., 17
Seitenwandleisten, 16
Semen, 65
Seminal vesicle(s), 20, 22, 41, 51, 58
"Semi-valvules," 7
Shaw, J. L., 126
Shoenberg, C. F., 76, 77
Shopfner, C. E., 27
Silverman, F. N., 142
"Sinovaginal bulbs," 16
Sinus, urogenital. *See* Urogenital sinus
"Sinus pocularis," 100
Sloane, J. A., 133
Smith, Blanca, 51
Smith, D. R., 24, 36, 149
Smith, J. C., 90
Smooth muscle(s), 19
  bundles of, 23, 24, 27, 28, 29, 30-55, 60
    in bladder, 65
    detrusor and, 24
    elastic fibers in, 61-63
    in the female, 46-48
    hypertrophy of, 122, 148
    in sphincteric urethra, 32f, 65

  of vesical neck, 31-33
  cellular morphology of, 76-85
  changes in, 5
  configuration of, 55
  contraction of, 81, 83, 85, 141
  degenerative disease of, 134
  detrusor and, 57f
  distensibility of, 141
  dysgenesis of, 133
  dysplasia of, 95, 142
  enzymatic studies of, 82
  excitation and, 82
  function of, in sphincteric urethra, 66, 67f
    in vesical neck, 66
  histological lesions in, 136-141, 137f, 138f
  hypertrophy of, 58, 94, 116, 163
  innervation and, 85
    nerves and, 73
  membranous urethra and, 41-45
  multi-unit, 79
  rhythmicity of, 74
  stimulation of, 80
  tone of, 95
  unitary, 80
  vacuolization of, 141
  vesical neck and, 45-46
Somatopleure, 133
Space of Retzius, 21
Spasm(s), bladder, 153
Specific gravity, urinary, 153
Sphincter(s), of Albarran, 45
  anal, 53, 66, 88, 166
    tone of, 155
  balance with detrusor of, 95, 131, 134
  external, 36, 49, 64, 80
  hypotonia of, 143-146
  innervation and, 73
  internal, 9, 25, 26, 27, 28, 36, 45, 80
  intrinsic striated, 38f, 40f, 42f, 43f, 46, 65, 75
    function and structure of, 65
  inhibition of, 69, 76
  resistance and, 86
  reduction of, 160
  striated external, electromyography of, 87
  urinary, 65
  urogenital, 41
"Sphincter internus," 9, 10
Sphincter trigonalis, 10
"Sphincter urethrae membranacae," 53
"Sphincter vesicae internus," 9
Sphincteric urethra, 90, 116, 146
  absence of, 166
  balance with detrusor of, 96

Sphincteric urethra (*Continued*)
  ballooning of, 150
  damage to, from instrumentation, 164
  development of, 11-19
  estimation of structure of, 156
  functions of, compromise of, 96
  gross anatomy of, 23-55
  histotopographic anatomy of, 30-55
  hypotonia of, 143
  innervation of, 48
  lesions of, 95, 97
  microscopic anatomy of, 55-63
  musculature of, 23-63, 34f, 37f
    intrinsic striated, 39-41
  paralysis of, 154
  polyps of, 96
  resistance of, 86, 122
  smooth muscle of, function of, 66, 67f
  smooth-muscle bundles in, 32f, 65
  stimulation of, 75
  tunica propria of, 55
  weakening of, 160
Spiking, action potentials and, 81
Spina bifida, 95
Spinal cord, 75, 131, 146
Sprunt, T. P., 100
Stain(s) and staining, 1, 59, 84, 135, 139
Stein, J., 134
Stenosis, membranous, 121
  pyloric, 8
  urethral meatus and, 149-150, 157
  valvular, 121
Stephens, F. D., 36, 88, 98, 100, 133
Sterling, A. M., 89
Stimulation, artificial electrical, 81
Stoesser, A. V., 143
Stohr, P., 51
Stone(s), formation of, 125
Straining, micturition and, 155
Stretch, 82
Submucosa, 55, 58
Succinic dehydrogenase, 82
Succinylcholine, 65
Sullivan, A. W., 94
Surgical procedure(s), 160, 161, 165.
  See also specific procedures
Suter, F., 125
Swaiman, K. F., 82, 135
Swenson, O., 133

TALIPES equinus, 142
Tambour(s), 89
Tanagho, E. A., 24, 36, 149
Teague, C. T., 80, 82

Telemetry, 86
"Tendoncillos," 33
Tension, measurement of, 86
Testicle(s), undescended, 95, 142
Testis(es), 143
Tetracaine, 79
Thaemert, J. C., 58, 76, 82
Thompson, G. J., 6
Thompson, G. S., 100
Tolmaltschew, H., 9, 100
Tone, anal sphincter and, 155
  bladder and, 134
Tonus, 69
  normal, 74
Trabeculation, 139, 146
Trabucco, A., 6
Training, 160, 165
Transducer(s), 86
Transmission, 80, 82
Transmitter release, 82
Transplantation, renal, 165
  ureteral, 166
Transurethral resection, 39, 94, 122, 159
Treatment, 94, 159-161. *See also*
  Management; Surgical procedure(s)
  further considerations in, 161-167
  sequence of, 159
Triad syndrome, 95, 133, 141-143, 145, 144f, 145f
Trigonal loop(s), 27, 28, 28f, 31, 35f, 45, 46, 66, 69, 75, 76, 105, 122
Trigone, 4, 14, 23, 31, 36, 39, 51, 55, 69, 95, 129, 142
  cells in, 73, 74, 74f
  erythema of, 164
  megacystis and, 131
  smooth muscle in, 65
  sympathetic innervation of, 64
Tropocollagen, 83
Tryptophan, 84
Tubercle(s), genital, 143
  Muller's, 15
Tumor(s), 150-151, 154
Tunica propria, 19, 28, 36, 51, 53, 55, 60, 74, 117, 120, 139, 148
  of sphincteric urethra, 55
Turbulence, 121
  urinary flow and, 90, 91
Tyrosine, 84

UHLENHUTH, E., 10, 23, 24, 26, 27, 30
Ulcer(s), meatal, 154
Ulceration, 149
Umbilicus, 15, 142, 153

Index 201

Unterkircher, Konrad, 107
Unterkircher anomaly, 107-115, 107f,
    109f, 110f, 111f, 112f, 113f, 114f
Urachus, 15, 23, 142
Uremia, 154
Ureter(s), 3, 13f, 15, 21, 143
    amount of muscle in, 135
    dilated, 145
    ectopic, 125
    function of, 80
    musculature of, 55
    tension in, 86
Ureteral colic, 153
Ureteral reflux, 91, 92, 95, 131, 132f,
    133, 145, 147, 156
Ureterocele(s), 125, 150, 159
Ureterosigmoidostomy, 166
Ureteroureterocutaneous anastomosis,
    166
Urethra, 15-19, 22
    atresia of, 4, 105
    bulbomembranous, 3, 39, 96, 143
        obstruction of, 103
    bulbous, 61, 73, 95, 102f, 125
        diverticula of, 96
    cavernous, 125
        stricture of, 96
    distal, 39
        lesions of, 97
    diverticula of, 125-126
    inframontane, 5, 18f, 39, 41, 45, 65,
        69, 73, 75, 99, 101f, 120
        elastic fibers in, 61
        obstruction of, 105
    membranous, 39, 44f, 48, 55, 66, 69,
        73, 75, 88, 98, 99, 120
        circular smooth muscle of, 41-45
        elastic fibers in, 61
    montane, 65
    musculature of, 19
    pendulous, 95, 125
    polyps of, 122-125, 124f
    posterior, 93, 145
    primary, 15, 17
    prostatic, 98
        cysts of, 96
    proximal, 66, 87
    resistance of, 156
    sphincteric. *See* Sphincteric urethra
    supramontane, 55
    tension in, 86
Urethral meatus, 19, 22, 24, 41, 87, 91,
    96, 105
    stenosis of, 149-150, 157
Urethral valves, 97-115
Urethrogram(s), voiding, 149

Urethrography, retrograde, 125, 159
Urethrovaginal septum, 31, 46
Urgency, urination and, 154
Urinary diversion, 165
Urinary flow, hydrodynamics of, 85-92
Urinary output, 153
Urination, 150. *See also* Micturition;
    Voiding
    control in inhibition of, 74
    cortical demand for, 75
    frequency of, 154
    initiation of, 65
    urgency of, 154
Urine, arrest of, 105
    exit velocity of, 87, 89
    odor and, 153, 154
    pink, 153
    red, 154
    residual. *See* Residual urine
    specific gravity of, 153
    transport of, 85
    turbulence of, 90, 91
Uroflowmetry, radioisotope, 92
Urogenital diaphragm, 19, 22, 53
    female, stress and strains on, 23
Urogenital sinus, 3, 11, 12f, 13, 14, 14f,
    15, 16, 16f, 19, 100, 103, 105, 107,
    125, 126, 166
    development of, 20f
    as origin of vaginal epithelium, 17
    radiography of, 159
    sarcoma of, 150
Urogram(s), intravenous, 164
Urography, 164
    intravenous, 155
Urorectal septum, 11, 12f
Uterus, 20
Utricle(s), 129
    prostatic, 17
"Utriculus," 100

VAGINA, 16, 16f, 17, 19, 103, 105, 129,
    154
    sarcoma of, 150
Vaginal cavity, 100
Vaginal reflux, 72f, 165
Vaginal septum, 41
Valve(s), 95, 103, 105, 116, 125
    resection of, 159
    urethral, 97-115
Valve leaflet(s), 100
van der Reis, L., 116
Vas deferens, 3, 20, 51, 58, 80, 155
Vein(s), hypogastric, 20
Velocity, urinary, 87, 89

Velpeau, A. A. L. M., 8
Vena contracta, 87, 89
Versari, R., 8, 10, 27, 31
  sphincter trigonalis of, 10
  vesicocervical fibers of, 8
Verumontanum, 8, 17, 19, 31, 33, 36, 39, 41, 55, 58, 60, 61, 69, 95, 98, 100, 123
  elastic fibers in, 116
  hypertrophy of, 96, 103
Vesical neck, 14f, 15, 22, 33, 36, 41, 65, 69
  abnormalities of, 94
  age-specific variations in, 5
  arterial supply to, 20
  cells in, 73
  contracture of, 116, 117
  cysts of, 96, 125
  as funnel, 69, 70f, 76, 90
  ganglia in, 49, 50, 50f
  glandular structure in, 55
  hypertrophy of, 8, 120-122
  mucosa in, 61
  nerve endings in, 74
  obstructions of, 96
    classification of, history of, 6-9
    history of, 5
    hypotheses of, 9-10
  opening of, 73
  plication of, 160
  resection of, 159
  retropubic approach to, 94
  smooth-muscle of, 31-33, 45-46
    function of, 66
  thickened, 147
  wide, 143
Vesicle(s), pinocytotic, 77
  presynaptic, 79
  postsynaptic, 79
  seminal, 20, 22, 41, 51, 58
Vestibule(s), 19, 24
Vilas, E., 17
Voiding. *See also* Micturition; Urination
  double, 165
  patterns of, 92
    disturbed, 91
  triple, 165
Voiding cystourethrogram(s). *See* Cystourethrogram(s), voiding
Vomiting, 153
Von Garrelts, B., 86, 87, 90, 91
Von Lichtenberg, A., 7
von Ludinghausen, H. J. F. H., 9, 10
Vulva, cleansing of, 165

WALDEYER, W., 9
Watson, E. M., 100
Wein, A. J., 82
Weinberg, S., 80, 134
Weinstein, H. J., 76
Wesson, M. B., 10, 24, 33
Whitaker, J., 87, 89
White, H., 88
Williams, D. I., 15, 125, 126, 131, 142, 145, 146, 150
Wilson, M. C., 94
Winckler, G., 55
Winter, C. C., 92
Wise, H. M., Jr., 7, 116
Wittus, W. S., 133
Wolffian duct(s), 9, 12, 15, 96, 100
Woodburne, R. T., 24, 26, 27, 28, 30, 33, 36, 65

YOUNG, B. W., 94, 117, 149
Young, H. H., 6, 7, 8, 24, 98, 100, 129
Y-V vesicourethroplasty, 94, 116, 117, 122, 160, 161f, 162f, 163f

ZANGMEISTER, W., 10
Zatz, I. M., 88, 89
Zinner, R., 89, 90

DATE DUE

NOV 27 1980			
APR 1 1992			
MAR 24 1992			

DEMCO 38-297